The Zen Days of Christmas

Christmas

**After All,
Who
Really Wants a
Partridge in a
Pear Tree?**

Carlene Snyder

ISBN-13: 978-1519711557
ISBN-10: 1519711557

The *Zen* Days of Christmas

After All, Who Really Wants a Partridge in a Pear Tree?

Table of Contents

The *Zen* Days of Christmas

Introduction

It's the most wonderful time of the year, or so the old song goes, but the sad reality is that for many, it is also the most stressful time of the year. The holiday hustle and bustle can leave us feeling cranky, tired, and out of sorts with life in general. It hits us on all levels, leaving us emotionally, physically, and financially drained. And if our own personal stresses aren't enough, because we are indeed connected by the Universal mind, what we experience is not only our own stress, but the stress of the entire collective consciousness as well. That very thought by itself is certainly enough to make you want to crawl back into bed and pull the covers up over your head and wait for the New Year.

But what if this year could be different? What if you could have a few tools in your tool belt (or shopping bag) that would help keep you physically, emotionally and spiritually balanced this season? We're faced with so many things *to do* that we forget that the season is really about giving and receiving love. We make it complicated, and in the complication we lose the joy. We become a human *doing* instead of a human *being*.

It's my hope that some of the suggestions in this book will allow you to navigate the holidays with less stress, more joy, and feeling your personal best. Wishing you all a very joyous and healthy holiday season filled to the brim with the simple joys of life.

The *Zen* Days of Christmas

On the **First** Day of Christmas, my Health Coach Gave to Me:

A Happy Holiday For Me

Christmas is that time of year that is filled with expectations, both of ourselves and of others, but do we really have a clear intention of how we'd like to approach the holiday? What can we start to do today that will allow us to experience the type of holiday season that our soul yearns for?

Well, first of all, let's take a look at the concept of intention. What exactly is intention and why it is important to get clear on this? Intention is that spark of energy that brings things from the world of thought into the world of reality. Without intention, our energy is scattered and we often lack the focus and persistence necessary to manifest what we desire in our lives. I like to view intention as our internal GPS system. We program in our intention and that intention directs our course of action in our day-to-day activities. When we find ourselves out of alignment in our lives, our internal GPS (our intention) recalculates to bring us back on course.

When you set an intention of what you would like to create for yourself, you allow yourself to focus in on that desired destination. That's not to say that you won't encounter some roads that have been washed out along the way, but if your intention is to get there, you can be assured that you will find a way.

So what are some practical steps that you can take in creating your intention and navigating the upcoming holiday with a sense of ease and purpose? Well here are some things you can do today, and every day to set and reach your destination.

Feel Your Intention as Your Current Reality - Spend some time each day, preferably first thing in the morning before you start your day, "feeling" what it would be like to achieve your intention. Bathe yourself in love, joy, peace, balance, and health. Imagine yourself experiencing the holidays filled with these emotions instead of feeling cranky, stressed, and fatigued. Allow yourself to really feel this reality in your body.

Create a Positive Affirmation - Create one or two positive affirmations based on the reality that you want to create. These affirmations should always be in the present tense, such as *I am peaceful and relaxed and am enjoying my holiday.* Or, *I feel blessed and grateful to be enjoying this holiday season in a way that honors my physical, emotional, and spiritual needs.*

Prioritize what matters - All too often we spend our energies on those things that don't matter. When we do this, we often neglect those very things in our life that *really* matter. We spend our time on things that don't support our ability to ever achieve our desires. For instance, if your intention is to have a holiday where you can enjoy time with your family, but you wait until the last minute to take care of the shopping, the cooking, and the decorating, how likely is it that you will realize your desire for a relaxed and enjoyable holiday? Instead of doing the things that will support you in achieving this reality, maybe you're spending most of your time on the computer or watching television. If that's the case, your actions are not in alignment with your intention. It's kind of like setting out on your trip without ever stopping to put gas in your car. You're going to run out of fuel along the way, making your chances of reaching your ultimate destination stressful at best.

Determine what means the most to you as you experience the holidays and then take the necessary action steps to achieve that goal. That might mean spending a weekend cooking and freezing some meals for when things get busy or getting that shopping out of the way right now. Also, take a look at what really needs to be done – not what you "think" needs to be done. Will the world stop if you don't send Christmas cards out this year? Do you really need to make six dozen different kinds of cookies? If you're doing things because you enjoy them, then great – that's a priority for you, but if you're doing it because you think it is "expected", then maybe you need to take a closer look.

Letting Go of the Need to Control - Holidays mean spending more time in close quarters with friends and family. While that sounds wonderful, the reality is that some of these folks may actually rub you the wrong way. What if you could let go of your need to control what other people think, do, or say? What if you didn't feel the need to judge the behavior of others or yourself? What if the judgment you feel from others didn't really matter to you anymore? What if you could just allow and be present? Holidays always bring out the opinions of others – especially the relatives. If someone pushes your buttons and you feel the need to give your opinion, maybe you could just listen, breathe, and smile instead and then gently redirect the conversation to something less charged. Letting go of the good opinions of others is a huge gift you can give to yourself. By releasing yourself from these judgments, you can remain on task, focusing on your personal intention, rather than being sucked into the drama of others. I'd like to give you an acronym to remember when you encounter challenging people or events that trigger an emotional response that doesn't align with your intention. David Gee, of the Chopra Center gives the acronym of **SODA** to walk you through a quick process of realignment when you encounter situations that bring out that desire to control.

> **S** – Stop. Notice that your emotions have been triggered.
> **O** – Observe. Notice what is going on around you. What do you see? What do you hear? What do you feel?

D – Detach. Pretend you're watching a movie. Release any expectation you may have regarding what is going on or your desired outcome. Imagine these thoughts as helium-filled balloons. Yep, there they are. The red one is irritation. Oh, and that blue one? That one is fear. Then imagine the balloons just floating off the screen while you're just seated there in your movie seat.

A – Awaken. Wake up to the present moment, because it is in this present moment that we accept what is and take action to manifest the future we desire. When we are truly awake, we can walk away from the drama and breathe in the contentment of remaining in our reality. Being present allows us to take the appropriate actions to stay with our intention.

Action Steps:

- Make multiple lists of your intention(s) and carry this list with you and post it in areas where you spend a significant amount of time each day. I like my refrigerator door in my kitchen or a Post-It Note on my computer. You can even create automatic calendar reminders that will pop up on a scheduled basis to remind you of your intention. Put a copy of your intention list by your bedside and refer to this list every night prior to bed and again first thing every morning. When you decorate for your holiday, buy one of those clear holiday balls and write your intention for this year on a tiny slip of paper and place it inside this ball. Every day that you see this ornament, let it remind you of your intention for this season.

- Now I realize that this next step may seem counter intuitive, but trust me, it is very necessary. Release this list of desires and intentions and surrender them to a higher power where creation occurs, trusting that when things don't seem to go the way you think they should, that there is a reason, and that the cosmic plan has designs much grander than any you could have ever envisioned.

- Remind yourself to practice present-moment awareness in all your actions. Refuse to allow obstacles to consume and dissipate the quality of your attention in the present moment. Accept the present as it is, and manifest the future through your deepest, most cherished intentions and desires.

So this holiday season set your intention to have a peaceful, joyous attitude. Look at all the ways you are blessed and supported in this life and set your intention to create this feeling as your own personal reality this year.

The *Zen* Days of Christmas

On the **Second** Day of Christmas, My Health Coach Gave to Me:

Two Loving Habits

Christmas is all about thinking of others and looking for ways to show the people in our lives how much we love and appreciate them. But all too often our own self care suffers in our desire to get things done, and we find ourselves entering the New Year not only feeling the exhaustion that Santa must experience, but kind of looking like him as well. A little extra padding without all the "ho ho ho". Quite possibly, Santa's jolly exterior is hiding months of working too hard and not getting adequate shut eye. All those late nights spent making toys, not to mention that one all-nighter spent delivering presents really doesn't look so merry and bright on those days following Christmas and leading up to the New Year. Is it any wonder that the first thing on many people's minds the beginning of the New Year is a detox or exercise program? Anyone can tell you that the local gym is sure to be packed come the first of the year.

So I'd like to suggest two loving habits to give yourself during the holidays that are simple and easy and will help you navigate the holidays feeling your best.

Loving Habit #1 – Sleep

The first loving habit you need to adopt for this season is - drum roll please – SLEEP! That's right, you're not going to be at your best if you short change yourself in the rest department. It has been shown that sleep deprivation directly impacts the health of your immune system, which means that if you're not getting enough sleep, you're increasing the likelihood of getting sick. Certainly not a gift you want to give yourself or others, especially during the holidays. Research also reveals that getting between seven and nine hours of sleep per night helps to reduce the body's response to stress, improves memory and cognitive function, and may even be beneficial to help you lose weight.

Besides, when you don't get enough shut-eye, you're more irritable, can't focus, and let's face it, just don't feel like yourself, which certainly doesn't put you in the holiday spirit. So, this year, make a commitment to get that required shut-eye every night. Here are some tips to help you achieve this goal:

- Get to bed by no later than 10 p.m. Everyone has a window of time when cortisol levels begins to dip and you feel tired. You need to catch this curve and get to bed when you start to feel tired. Otherwise, if you push through it, you will have missed the curve and you'll catch a second cortisol spike that will make it hard to relax and go to sleep. Traditional Chinese Medicine believes that it is imperative to be in bed with eyes closed by 11 p.m., as it is between the hours of 11 p.m. to 3 a.m. that the gallbladder and liver work on detoxifying your body. It's kind of like when you work late and the janitorial staff shows up to clean your office and there you are, still working away. They can't do their work because you're right in their way. You need to be gone in order for them to really clean your office and empty the trash. Otherwise, they skip your cubicle and you come back the next morning to a dirty office. When your liver comes to clean up, you need to be off in dreamland.
- Spend at least one hour before bedtime electronics free. That's right – no television, computer work, emails, etc. one hour prior to bed. You'll just have to

Facebook your friends or watch that funny cat video at another time.

- When the computer goes off, it's also time to dim the lights. Bright lights keep the body from producing melatonin, a hormone that signals the brain that it's time for sleep. So rather than having so many lights on, consider turning most of them off and just have a little relaxing mood lighting instead. Hey, it's Christmas, so dim the normal lighting and just enjoy the twinkle of the holiday lights on the tree – that is unless you're Chevy Chase and have your halls decked to the point where your neighbors start to complain. In the bedroom, make sure it is dark – no outside ambient light or lights from electronic devices. Keep the bedroom for sleeping and make it an electronics-free zone.

- Exercise during the day. People who make exercise a part of their lifestyle sleep better. So try to find a time of day that works best for you. For some, exercising in the morning works, or maybe a walk during your lunch hour or after work. For some folks, exercising in the morning is the best, as they find that exercise too close to bedtime makes it difficult for them to relax, while others find exercising later in the day helps them unwind. Find out what is true for you and exercise accordingly.

- Limit caffeine, alcohol, and nicotine. Alcohol may seem to relax you but will disrupt your sleep later in the night. Keep the caffeine to a minimum, I'd suggest no more than 1-2 small cups a day, and drink it before lunch. Nicotine is a stimulant and isn't a habit you want to keep for many reasons; a good night's rest is one of them.

- Get some light during the day. If you can get outside and enjoy the natural sunshine, great. If not, consider investing in a "Happy Light" and exposing yourself to some morning light. Light exposure during the day is important in regulating the circadian rhythm and can make a difference for falling asleep at night.

- Keep the electronics out of the bedroom. This is NOT, I repeat NOT YOUR OFFICE! Keep the bedroom associated with sleeping and intimacy only – no work or TV.

- Make sure your bed is large enough and is comfortable, and invest in good pillows that support the alignment of your neck and spine. And while I love my pets, our furry little friends can be disruptive to your sleep. I have a cat that snores and another one that runs in and out of my vertical blinds all night. So giving them their own beds is imperative to me getting my rest.

- Keep your bedroom on the cool side. Studies show that the optimal room temperature for sleep is quite cool, between 60 to 68 degrees (16-20 Celsius). Keeping your room cooler or hotter than this can lead to restless sleep.

- If you can't get away from noise, install some white noise from an air cleaner or similar source. This will cover the other noise and not interfere with sleep.

- Consider wearing socks on your feet. If you're like me, my feet get very cold – especially in the winter. Keeping your feet warm can help improve circulation in your extremities, which can help you fall asleep more quickly.

- Consider a little aromatherapy. I love the calming effect of essential oils. Diffusing lavender, sage, valerian, vetiver, roman chamomile, sandalwood, and marjoram are great oils to reduce anxiety and stress. You can also mix a few drops of essential oils with some coconut oil and rub this mixture on the bottoms of your feet, then put on some socks and go to bed.

- Consider hiding your alarm clock. How many times do you wake up during the night and try to see what time it is? For me, this is difficult, as my alarm clock is across the room, and without my glasses I can't see it, so why bother? What you end up doing when you're trying to see the time is stressing yourself out, which makes it even more difficult to fall back to sleep. Consider moving your alarm clock across the room and away from you, and placing a small hand towel over the clock. When it goes off, you will then need to get out of bed to shut it off, and the temptation to keep hitting that snooze bar won't be happening.

- Try to establish a regular schedule for your sleep. Go to bed at the same time and wake up at the same time every day. If you nap, take your naps earlier in the afternoon and keep them short. Sometimes a 30-minute power nap can do wonders, but if you sleep for hours, you may not be able to fall asleep at night.

- Incorporate bedtime rituals. Listen to music, take a warm bath, drink a cup of herbal tea and read a few minutes in the evening to unwind, but maybe skip the murder mysteries this time of night.

Loving Habit #2 – Stay Hydrated

When the weather gets cooler, we often don't think about keeping ourselves as hydrated. But in the winter, it's just as important to make sure that you're getting enough water.

For one thing, if you're dehydrated, you're more likely to think that you're hungry, and the holiday season has food available at every turn. Keeping yourself well hydrated will make the temptation to eat more calorically dense foods less likely.

Proper hydration also will provide you with better energy during the day. Lack of hydration will leave you feeling droopy. Imagine what happens to a plant when it doesn't receive enough water. Make sure that you have a water bottle handy in the car, at your office, and at home and keep the fluids going. You will need your energy during this season to feel your best.

There's some disagreement on how much water a person needs, but I always encourage people to start their day by drinking a glass of water, as this is the time of day that you're the most dehydrated. Also, drinking at least two glasses of water between meals is a good practice to incorporate, but limit fluid intake at mealtimes. Many people don't produce adequate amounts of hydrochloric acid, which is needed to properly digest your food, so drinking large amounts of water at mealtimes can dilute these digestive fluids.

Listen to your body, and if you find hunger pangs starting up between meals, try drinking a large glass of water and waiting for about 20 minutes to see if that is what your body needed instead of looking for that snack.

Try Warm Lemon Water – So I'm giving you a little bonus here, but it goes along with the hydration tip. When my digestive system started to bother me, I had to give up drinking coffee in the morning, and I won't lie to you, this was one sad girl. There was just something about holding that warm cup in my hand first thing in the morning. Honestly, I think I enjoyed the smell of the coffee almost as much as the taste, and, in fact, I didn't really enjoy the flavor of the coffee so much – I think it was all the cream and sugar, but that's a topic for another day.

So, how did I cut out coffee while my gut healed? Enter warm lemon water.

What I realized was that my stomach needed a little extra acid so that I could digest my food, and guess what works to increase stomach acid? That's right - lemon! In addition to giving digestion a boost, it also hydrates the body. When we wake up in the morning, our body has gone without water for hours and is very dehydrated. So instead of throwing a liquid like coffee into your system, which will further dehydrate your body, try warm lemon water.

Traditional Chinese Medicine and Ayurvedic philosophy both believe that that the daily choices we make can either strengthen the body or deplete the body of essential life force. Adopting this simple habit sets your body up for the remainder of the day. Some of the benefits of drinking the warm lemon water are as follows:

- **Boosts the immune system** - Lemons are high in vitamin C and potassium. Vitamin C is great for fighting colds and potassium stimulates brain and nerve function and helps control blood pressure.
- **Balances pH** - Lemons are an incredibly alkaline food. Yes, they are acidic on their own, but inside our bodies they're alkaline (the citric acid does not create acidity in the body once metabolized).
- **Helps with weight loss** - Lemons are high in pectin fiber, which helps fight hunger cravings. It also has

been shown that people who maintain a more alkaline diet lose weight faster.

- *Aids digestion* - The warm water serves to stimulate the gastrointestinal tract and peristalsis - the waves of muscle contractions within the intestinal walls that keep things moving. Lemons are also high in minerals and vitamins and help loosen toxins in the digestive tract.

- *Acts as a gentle, natural diuretic* - Lemon juice helps flush out unwanted materials because lemons increase the rate of urination in the body. As a result, toxins are released more quickly, helping keep your urinary tract healthy.

- *Clears skin* - Who doesn't want to look their best at those holiday parties? The vitamin C from the lemon helps decrease wrinkles and blemishes. Lemon water purges toxins from the blood which helps keep skin clear as well.

- *Supports Adrenal Function* - When your body is dehydrated it can't perform properly, which leads to toxic buildup, stress, constipation, and the list just goes on. Your adrenals happen to be two small glands that sit on top of your kidneys, and along with your thyroid, create energy. They also secrete important hormones, including aldosterone. Aldosterone is a hormone secreted by your adrenals that regulates water levels and the concentration of minerals, like sodium, in your body, helping you stay hydrated. Your adrenals are also responsible for regulating your stress response. The adrenal glands thrive on vitamin C from the lemons, so not only are you hydrating the body, you're giving your adrenal glands a little vitamin C as well.

If you're concerned about the lemon water harming tooth enamel, you can always sip the water through a straw. There are some great glass straws that can be purchased that eliminate the concern of drinking through plastic straws if you're concerned about either environmental considerations or the toxic exposure from plastics. Try this habit for a month and don't be surprised if you find a new habit that you will want to stay with. The recipe isn't complicated – just a cup of warm water and the juice from half of a lemon. Simple and easy – just what you need during the hectic holiday season.

The *Zen* Days of Christmas

On the **Third** Day of Christmas My Health Coach Gave to Me:

Three Grateful Thoughts

If there was one specific thing I could tell you to do each day that would change your life, would you do it? Well friends, write this one down, because this one is most definitely a game changer. It's gratitude! Yes, being thankful and grateful for the blessings you currently have, not to mention those that are already on their way to you, is one of the most important things you can do. Now, I'm just not talking about saying, "I am grateful for my house", or "I am grateful for my children". That's great, but I want you to go deeper. Really give some thought to your blessings. Feel your heart expand with love and true appreciation. Experience the true blessing that you feel deep down in your soul.

Gratitude, like love, is a high-frequency emotion, and staying in this vibration has a very direct correlation with bringing more of this high vibrational energy into your life. The more thankful you are, the more positive circumstances will show up for you. Every-where we turn today, we hear about how damaging stress is to our health. Well folks, negative thoughts ARE stress, and the more you choose to dwell on what isn't working for you, the more these neg-ative thoughts impact your body, mind, and spirit. What you choose to think about is your choice, so choose grateful thoughts. Once you understand that you are the master of your stress levels, and that by choosing thoughts of gratitude you can actually decrease stress, you then become the creator of more positive life experiences.

Here's another twist I'd like you to try. If you're trying to change something in your life, for instance, if you want to lose weight, feel grateful that you have accomplished your goal. That's right; spend some time in gratitude for this desire as if it has already happened for you. Thank your body for all the amazing ways it supports you. Even say out loud, "I wonder why it was so *EASY* for me to lose weight and keep my weight stable?"

Want to take gratitude to a whole new level? Begin by being grateful for the things in your life that aren't perfect. For years I suffered with severe digestive issues, and I would get down on my knees every night and pray for them to go away. If there had been a magic Genie that would grant me a wish, this would have been my wish. But that chronic pain was one of the biggest blessings in my life. This pain moved me to take action on things I could change in my life, which led me down an alternative path to health and healing.

I truly believe that when we look at things in our life with gratitude, we send this high vibrational energy out into the ethers, and in turn, our own personal experiences are enriched.

I was listening to Joyce Meyer on television one day and she was teaching on gratitude. She told a story where a child came to the parent and wanted new shoes. The parent said, "I realize you want new shoes, and I will find some time to make sure you get them." Then she presented two possible ways the child could react. In one scenario, the child would whine every day that they were never going to get new shoes, and in the second scenario, the child would excitedly anticipate that they were going to get new shoes, expressing gratitude to the parents that these new shoes were on their way. Her conclusion was this - if you're this parent, wouldn't you really want to get that excited, grateful child the shoes as soon as possible?

Action Steps:

Here's something that is easy to do and is a great family project as well. This could also be a wonderful DIY Christmas present to give to a friend. Create a Gratitude Jar. It doesn't have to be anything fancy – a mason jar will do, or a large bowl will work as well. I found a jar at Ikea and decorated it with some colorful stickers and found some cards to write my blessings on. You can even print off your items on your computer and put them in the jar. Maybe it's a picture of someone you love. Just print it off and write on the back of the picture why you are grateful for this person.

Each day, I want you to pick three things for which you feel grateful. Write them on a slip of paper and spend a few moments, close your eyes, and focus in on the gratitude you feel. Try to find something new each day. It might be as simple as a cup of coffee or a smile from a stranger.

Then on another sheet of paper, or on the back of your previous note, write down something that hasn't happened yet, but that you would really like in your life. Now, express gratitude for this and spend some time feeling this as a reality in your life. Experience the excitement and joy, then put this paper in the jar and release this desire to the field of infinite possibilities.

If you can't come up with three things each day, just do the best you can. You can do this throughout the course of the holiday season through the end of the year. Then on New Year's Eve, open up the jar and count your blessings. The idea is to get you and your family vibrating at that higher frequency of gratitude.

The *Zen* Days of Christmas

On the **Fourth** Day of Christmas, My Health Coach Gave to Me:

Four Deep Breaths

I learned of this breathing exercise from Andrew Weil, M.D., and he refers to it as the 4:7:8 Breath, or Relaxing Breath. It is super simple, takes almost no time, requires no special equipment and can be done anywhere. Although you can do the exercise in any position, sit with your back straight while learning the exercise.

Place the tip of your tongue against the ridge of tissue just behind your upper front teeth, and keep it there through the entire exercise. You will be exhaling through your mouth around your tongue. Try pursing your lips slightly if this seems awkward.

- Exhale completely through your mouth, making a whoosh sound.
- Close your mouth and inhale quietly through your nose to a mental count of four.
- Hold your breath for a count of seven.
  Exhale completely through your mouth, making a whoosh sound to a count of eight. (Exhalation should take twice as long as the inhalation.)
- This is one breath. Now inhale again and repeat the sequence three more times for a total of four complete cycles.
- That's it! Do it at *least* twice a day. You cannot do it too frequently. Do not do more than four breaths at one time for the first month of practice. Later, if you wish, you can extend it to eight breaths. You may feel

a little lightheaded when you first breathe this way, but this should soon pass.

The absolute time you spend on each phase is not important; the ratio of 4:7:8 is what matters. If you have trouble holding your breath, speed up the exercise, but keep to the ratio of 4:7:8 for the three phases. With practice you can slow it all down and get used to inhaling and exhaling more and more deeply.

This exercise is a natural tranquilizer for the nervous system. While it is very subtle when you begin, it gains power with repetition and practice. Use the 4:7:8 breath whenever anything upsetting happens – before you react, or when you're aware of internal tension. It is recommended to be used to help you fall asleep or to control cravings.

The *Zen* Days of Christmas

On the **Fifth** Day of Christmas, My Health Coach Gave to Me:

Five Super Foods

The stress of the holiday season can often leave our diet chaotic and hit and miss at best. If you're not eating well, you're not feeling well, so finding easy ways to get some healthy foods into your diet is imperative for keeping your system running smoothly, especially when we all have so many extra things on our plate. The last thing anyone wants this time of the year is to get run down and sick. An unexpected cold can send your energy and spirit plummeting and can definitely take the merry out of your Christmas. Enter the Five Superfoods that you might want to consider adding into your daily repertoire to keep you happy and healthy during the holiday season.

Superfood #1 - Wild Blueberries

In the world of fruits, wild blueberries are not only delicious, they're a powerful antioxidant. Wild blueberries are rich in the flavonoid anthocyanin, which protects against the effects of free radicals in the body, guarding it against disease and the effects of aging. Anthocyanin pigments give blueberries their deep color and are concentrated in the skin of the berries. Since the wild blueberries are much smaller, there are more of these anthocyanins concentrated in the same amount, cup for cup, compared to cultivated blueberries.

Among other health benefits, they are great for the skin. They support the skin's collagen, prevent wrinkling, decrease cellulite, fight bruising, and minimize acne breakouts. If want your skin looking great for those holiday parties, don't forget the wild blueberries this year. They are simple to add into your morning smoothie or are great sprinkled on your morning oatmeal.

Wild Blueberry Fruit Salad

Ingredients:

2 packages (6 ounces each) Wild Blueberries
1 cup pomegranate seeds
¼ cup sunflower seeds
¼ cup pumpkin seeds
¼ cup slivered, toasted almonds
¼ cup unsweetened coconut
Pinch of cinnamon
1 - 2 tsp. honey

Method:

Place all ingredients in a bowl and toss thoroughly to coat with the honey.

Superfood #2 – Avocados

If you're a fan of that creamy texture on your tongue, then let me introduce you to the avocado. I have been known to turn these little green gems into chocolate pudding. My oldest granddaughter, Lilly, once told me when she was just a toddler that she didn't like avocados. I believe she said "I no like avocados, Grandma." I still remember the disgusted look on her adorable face and her little wrinkled-up nose as I was putting them into my shopping cart. I then asked her if she liked chocolate pudding, to which she enthusiastically replied, "YES!" I then proceeded to tell her that Grandma was able to magically turn avocados into chocolate pudding. Even as a toddler, she wasn't easy to convince, but after I tossed a few other ingredients into the food processor and let it spin it's magic, I had even this skeptical child hooked. Wha Lah! Introducing chocolate pudding, which was greeted with an eager spoon and a chocolate grin.

And why wouldn't you fall in love with this super food? Avocados are an excellent source of folate, vitamins C, K, E, and B6 as well as calcium, copper, iron, phosphorous and magnesium. In fact, avocados contain more potassium than bananas.

People are often concerned because they believe that avocados are high in fat, but it's a healthy monounsaturated fat and has been shown to actually improve a person's cholesterol by reducing the bad (LDL) cholesterol and increasing the good (HDL) cholesterol. Additionally, the fats in avocados have been shown to reverse insulin resistance by helping to steady blood sugar levels. They contain oleic acid, an important nutrient that helps our digestive tract transport fat molecules that increase our absorption of fat-soluble nutrients. Avocados also have been shown to protect again breast cancer and slow the growth of prostate cancer. And since they contain more lutein than other common fruits, avocados protect the eyes against cataracts and macular degeneration.

A great source of the immune booster, glutathione, avocados help keep the heart and nervous system strong as well as slow the aging process.

Slice up an avocado and include it in your morning smoothie for extra creaminess. Your morning eggs are extra special topped with a sliced avocado and salsa, and there's no better accompaniment to Mexican food than a side of homemade guacamole. Instead of a bowl of chips and dip, make up a batch of guacamole and have some raw veggies available for dipping. And if your sweet tooth needs a new treat, try the chocolate avocado pudding recipe below:

Chocolate Avocado Pudding

Ingredients:

2 large or 3 small avocados

½ cup plus 2 Tbs. real maple syrup

2 tsp. vanilla

1 tsp. balsamic vinegar

½ tsp. gluten-free tamari sauce (soy sauce)

2 Tbs. coconut concentrate or coconut oil

3-4 pitted dates (chopped)

⅓ cup of cacao powder

Sliced strawberries or raspberries (optional for topping)

Method:

Cut the avocados in half and scoop out the meat. Slice into chunks and place in the food processor. Add the chopped pitted dates, maple syrup, vanilla, balsamic vinegar, tamari sauce, coconut concentrate or coconut oil. Process until somewhat smooth. Add the cacao powder and continue processing until texture is smooth and creamy. Chill mixture in the refrigerator until cold. Slice strawberries into small serving cups and add a dollop of chocolate pudding. Top with a few slices of strawberries, raspberries, or other fresh fruit of your choice. For an added indulgence, whip up some cashew nut cream sauce to drizzle on top of your pudding.

Cashew Nut Cream Sauce

Ingredients:

½ cup raw cashews

2-3 Tbs. maple syrup

1 tsp. vanilla

2-3 Tbs. of water

Method:

In a high-speed blender (I use my Vitamix), place cashews, maple syrup, water and vanilla and blend until smooth and creamy. I typically soak the cashews for a few hours prior to making the sauce, making them softer and easier to process. This sauce is also wonderful drizzled over fresh fruit (I love it with apples or berries).

Superfood #3 - Camu Camu Powder

The camu berry is possibly something new to you. This berry comes from the Amazon rainforest and is best known for its unusually high vitamin C content. Because vitamin C is a powerful antioxidant, it prevents free radical damage to our DNA and provides numerous health benefits to the body.

There's no food on the planet with a higher concentration of vitamin C than the camu berry. Camu Camu (it's so good they have to say it twice) has almost 30 times more vitamin C than your average orange. It also contains vitamin B3 and potassium. Vitamin B3 helps with the energy production of the cells and maintains the healthy functioning of the nervous and digestive systems. It also contains potassium, a mineral that helps promotes the proper functioning of the brain, heart, and muscles in the body.

I purchase raw organic Camu Camu powder from Sunfood, and one teaspoon of this powder states it supplies 240 percent of the RDA of vitamin C. Since your body is constantly eliminating vitamin C, I find that putting just a bit of this powder in my drinking water lets me replenish this nutrient throughout the day. There are many other manufacturers of Camu Camu powder, so just do your research and make sure you are purchasing a quality product that is organic and doesn't contain added ingredients.

Here's a list of some of Camu Camu's virtues:

- **Boosts the Immune System** - This helps fight off those seasonal colds and flu bugs.
- **Helps Neutralize Pollutants** - Let's face it, we live in a world filled with toxins, so any help we can get to mitigate this exposure is something to incorporate daily.
- **Maintains Healthy Organs** – Camu Camu reduces plaque buildup in the brain and arteries, supports healthy eye function, and maintains the overall health of the nervous system.
- **Natural Antihistamine** – If you suffer from seasonal allergies, Camu Camu can reduce some of these symptoms.
- **Anti-Inflammatory** – As a natural anti-inflammatory, Camu Camu can reduce the body's inflammatory response, which in turn can help those who experience arthritis pain.
- **Anti-Viral** – Camu Camu has been shown to be powerful in preventing and controlling the herpes virus. In *The Clinician's Handbook of Natural Healing*, Gary Null, Ph.D. rates Camu Camu at the top of the list of 19 plants that contain anti-herpetic phytochemicals.
- **Anti-Depressant** – According to *New Help for Depression* by Elora Gabriel, the camu berry is one of the natural strategies you can use to reverse depression. So if the holidays aren't always the best time of year for you, this added boost might be something for you to consider.
- **Fights Migraines** – Camu Camu has also been shown to be helpful for people who suffer from headaches and migraines, especially those headaches

that result from toxicity of any kind (internal or external).

You can add this powder into juices, smoothies, and even your water. The powder doesn't always dissolve well, so I often just put my water into my NutriBullet, add the powder and blend it for just a minute, but you certainly don't need to do this. A quick stir with a spoon works just as well, or one of those little shaker bottles could also work. You can add Camu Camu to things like applesauce or cooked fruits or yogurts for a little extra tang.

Here's a quick and healthy dessert that you can easily pull together that incorporates this superfood:

Mango Yogurt Sorbet

Ingredients:
2 cups frozen chunked organic mango
1 tsp. Camu Camu powder
1 container yogurt (I used coconut milk yogurt)
½ cup water
4 tsps. honey
Dash of cinnamon and ginger (optional). It's good with or without the spices.

Method:
Place all ingredients in high-speed blender and process until smooth. Serve immediately.

Now, if all the things I've told you about Camu Camu doesn't have you heading out to get some, here's one more way to use it to keep you glowing this holiday season. You can make your own skin care cleansers and serums using this powder. I make a cleanser that is basically a little bit of honey and a sprinkle of Camu Camu powder. Basically, I just stir this together and wash my face with it.

You can also create a natural Vitamin C serum to put on your face. I discovered an online recipe from www.hellonatural.co for making your own serum.

Vitamin C Skin Serum

Ingredients:
4 teaspoons aloe vera gel
2 teaspoons glycerin
2 teaspoons Camu Camu powder

Method:
Combine Camu Camu and glycerin and mix well. Add aloe vera and stir to combine. Transfer to small container (one with a dropper is the easiest to use).

To use, smooth 2-4 drops onto (clean) face, neck and chest twice a day. Let it absorb and follow with moisturizer.

Superfood #4 – Tumeric

Turmeric, aka *curcumin*, is a powerful anti-inflammatory and antioxidant. You can purchase it as a spice and it is also available in capsule form so you can take it as a supplement.

Tumeric has been shown to be effective in the treatment of inflammatory bowel disease and is helpful for reducing inflammation for those with arthritis. It is thought to prevent cancer, improve cardiac function, lower cholesterol, and fight depression. Additionally, it has been found to be helpful in the treatment of Alzheimer's.

It has been shown that adding black pepper along with turmeric increases the bioavailability of the turmeric by up to 2000%!

So, what are some quick and easy ways to incorporate turmeric into your diet? You can easily mix up your own healthy curry powder that you can throw into any vegetable stir-fry, cooked lentils, egg salad, scrambled eggs or scrambled tofu.

Curry Powder Recipe

Ingredients:
2 Tbs. ground coriander
2 Tbs. ground cumin
1 Tbs. tumeric powder
1 tsp. ground black pepper
½ tsp. ground mustard seeds
½ tsp. ground ginger

Method:
Mix these spices together and store in a jar. I recommend that you use organic spices when putting this mix together. You can save money buying these spices from the bulk bins at your natural health food store, purchasing small amounts in the quantities you need.

Another thing you might enjoy is turmeric tea.

Creamy Tumeric Tea

Ingredients:
1 cup almond or coconut milk
½ tsp. turmeric
½ -inch slice of ginger root, peeled and finely chopped
¼ tsp. ground ginger
Dash of cayenne pepper

½ – 1 tsp. honey
Optional additions: a small pat of butter, cinnamon, or cardamom

Method:
Gently warm the almond or coconut milk on the stove. In a mug, combine the remaining ingredients.

Drizzle a teaspoon of the warmed milk into the mug and mix until the liquid is smooth with no lumps. Add the rest of the milk and mix well. You can leave the pieces of ginger in the tea, or strain it out before drinking.

Superood #5 – Kale

Kale is one of my staple foods. I like the curly kind and the "dino" kale. Kale is low in calories (about 33 calories per cup) and a great source of vitamins A, C, and K, as well as beta-carotene, which are all important co-factors and antioxidants. It's also a decent source of calcium and manganese. For some people, raw kale can be tough to digest, so don't forget that you can cook with it as well which will help with digestion. Cooking kale doesn't alter the antioxidant benefits.

If you tolerate it raw, throw it into your smoothies or make a massaged kale salad with olive oil, sea salt and a little lemon. You can also sauté it in avocado oil, ghee, or butter with salt, pepper and spices like cumin, coriander and nutmeg. Sprinkle it with Parmesan cheese and raw pumpkin seeds, and add diced pears or figs for a little natural sweetness. You can also lightly coat the leaves with avocado oil and sea salt and stick them under the broiler for a few seconds to make kale chips. Here's my favorite recipe for kale chips:

Kale Chips

Ingredients:
1 large bunch of curly, green kale washed, large stems removed, torn into bite size pieces

Coating:
1 cup cashews (soaked 2 hours)
1 red bell pepper, seeded and chopped
Juice of 1 lemon
1 Tbs. nutritional yeast
¼ tsp. garlic or onion powder
½ tsp. Himalayan pink crystal salt (use more or less to taste)
Options: If you like yours spicy, add in some jalapeno pepper or you can also add some of your favorite salsa.

Method: Put coating ingredients in a high-speed blender (I use my Vitamix) and blend until smooth.

Place torn kale leaves into a large bowl, and using your hands, massage coating and kale pieces together, getting the coating inside of all the curls on the kale leaves. Put coated leaves on the parchment paper on two large baking sheets. (Don't worry about flattening them, they're better bunched up) and place in your oven at its lowest temperature (mine goes down to 170 degrees). You might want to crack open the door to your oven to allow steam to escape for the first hour or so of baking. If you happen to own a food dehydrator, this is probably the preferred method to make these chips. Just let them dehydrate about 10 hours, or until dry.

Or, if you're like me and only have an oven, just bake until crispy on your oven's lowest setting (approximately 3-4 hours). You might want to flip the chips over at some point to facilitate the drying process. Cool and store in an airtight container.

The *Zen* Days of Christmas

On the **Sixth Day** of Christmas, My Health Coach Gave to Me:

Six Slimming Smoothies

Smoothies are a quick and easy way to pack a bunch of nutrition into a portable meal. Let's face it, the holidays are often busy, so we're all looking for ways to get something quick, but we'd like to keep those empty calories under control.

Smoothies are a great way to get in some healthy plant protein, fruits and veggies, and once you get the hang of it, you can even bag contents for your smoothies together ahead of time and freeze individual smoothie bags. Just a few minutes of filling up some quart-size freezer bags can give you a head start with including more fruits and veggies into your diet during this holiday season. When you're ready for a smoothie, just reach in your freezer and pull one of these freezer bags out, empty the contents into your blender, and add your liquid of choice. I even found that Costco has an organic smoothie mix (mixed berries and kale) individually packed so that's another time-saving option if you can find this already done for you. Costco's blend was a little slim on the kale, but for the person just starting out with smoothies, it's a great place to start.

In order to streamline the process and give you an idea of what you need in your smoothies, here's a simple breakdown:

1) **Fruits** - Buy some big bags of frozen fruit, or if you have fresh fruit, that works too. I like to include a fresh fruit like an apple or pear because you can't find them frozen, but you can certainly prep and freeze some of your own.

2) **Liquid** - Get some liquid staples to have on hand like coconut milk, rice milk, almond milk, hemp milk, or co-

conut water and put these in your pantry. Remember filtered water works as well.

3) **Protein** - Buy a container of quality organic pea, rice, or hemp protein powder that you like, or buy a bag of hemp seeds or chia seeds, or seed or nut butters. Or if you like yogurt, freeze individual portions of yogurt (coconut yogurt works if you're dairy free) in ice cube trays. This is the protein part of your smoothie.

4) **Vegetables** – Buy cartons of pre-washed spinach or kale or other leafy greens that you like. You can also pick up other veggies such as cucumbers, carrots or celery and prep those for your bags.

5) **Spices** – Pick up some organic spices that you like. Some of my favorites are ginger and cinnamon.

6) **Container** - Buy some quart-size Ziploc bags and assemble everything but the liquid into the bags. A simple ratio to follow is:

- 1 soft fruit (pear, apple, banana, or ½ an avocado)
- 1 cup frozen fruit (blueberries, raspberries, strawberries, mangos, pineapple, or mixed berry blends work really well)
- 1 to 2 Tbs. of protein powder, hemp seeds, chia seeds, or nut butters. You can also take Greek yogurt or coconut yogurt and pre-freeze them in an ice cube tray, and put a few of these into the bag with the fruits. Or, if you don't have an ice cube tray, simply put the yogurt into a zip lock bag, cut a small hole in the end, and pipe little yogurt dots onto parchment paper on a

small baking sheet and place this in your freezer until they are solid.

- 1 to 1½ cups of greens or a mix of greens with
other vegetables such as cucumber or celery.
Chop them up into small pieces so that they will
blend easily. If you'd like to pre-blend your
greens and veggies, you can blend them up and
then freeze them in ice cube trays as well and
just pop them in with your frozen fruit in your
smoothie bag. I'd suggest using about 3 cubes
of greens tossed in with your frozen fruit. One
of the smaller pre-washed containers of greens
(5 ounces), blended with a small amount of water makes one full ice cube tray for me.

It doesn't get any easier than that. I've tried to keep these
smoothies super simple, just a few ingredients, but use your own
creativity and feel free to include those other ingredients that you
have on hand that work for you and your own personal taste. Don't
forget including some of the superfoods from the previous chapter.
They all work great in smoothies.

#1 - Wild Blueberry, Pear, and Celery Smoothie
Ingredients:
½ to 1 cup of frozen wild blueberries
1 stalk celery (chunked)
1 pear (chunked)
1-2 scoops of your favorite rice or pea protein powder

Method:

Combine all ingredients in the blender and add enough water to cover the ingredients. Blend until smooth.

#2 - Holiday Bloat Blaster Smoothie

Ingredients:

½ cup coconut water
1 banana
1 small cucumber, sliced and chunked
1 inch piece of fresh ginger, peeled and sliced
Handful of ice

Method:

Combine all ingredients in the blender and blend until smooth.

#3 - Strawberries and Cream Smoothie

Ingredients:

1 heaping cup of frozen strawberries
1 frozen banana (chunked)
1 cup almond milk or coconut milk
1 tsp. honey or maple syrup
½ tsp. vanilla extract (optional)

Method:

Place all ingredients in a blender and blend until smooth. Feel free to add protein powder for an added boost of protein.

#4 - Mango, Coconut and Chia Seed Smoothie
Ingredients:

8 pieces of frozen mango (about ¾ cup)

½ cup coconut milk

1 Tbs. chia seeds

2 Tbs. shredded, unsweetened coconut

¼ tsp. ground nutmeg or cinnamon

1 scoop protein powder

Method:

Place frozen mango, coconut milk, and protein powder in blender and blend until smooth. Add in chia seeds and pulse to combine. Top with unsweetened coconut and a sprinkle of cinnamon or nutmeg.

#5 – Mint Chocolate Smoothie
Ingredients:

¼ cup avocado, mashed

¼ cup vanilla Greek yogurt or vanilla coconut yogurt

2 Tbs. vanilla protein powder

1 Tbs. honey or maple syrup

¼ tsp. peppermint extract

¾ cup unsweetened almond milk

1 tsp. vanilla extract

½ cup kale, firmly packed

½ cup ice

1 Tbs. chocolate chips (I like the Enjoy Life brand)

Method:

Blend all ingredients until smooth.

#6 – Tropical Oasis Smoothie

Ingredients:

2 cups spinach

1 orange (peeled)

1 cup coconut water

1 cup pineapple

1 banana

Method:

Blend ingredients in a high-speed blender until smooth.

The *Zen* Days of Christmas

On the **Seventh Day** of Christmas, My Health Coach Gave to Me:

Seven Simple Suppers

We're so busy during the holidays planning for holiday meals and parties that we often find ourselves short on time to put a healthy meal on our own dinner table. This is where simplicity steps in. Things need to be quick, healthy, comforting, and easy. One of the first things I learned in health coaching was that it was easier for people to cook once and eat twice. Personally, while I sometimes enjoy cooking, I can get worn out being in the kitchen, especially when my "to do" list is full of unchecked items. I've also found that it is nice to have some healthy meals in the freezer ready to go for those days when I'm either just not in the mood to spend a lot of time in the kitchen, or there are other things that I'd rather spend my time on. If you're already going to be spending time prepping a meal, just double the recipe for the main course and put another meal in the freezer for another day. Then stock up on some pre-washed organic salad mixes, frozen vegetables, fresh vegetables and fresh fruit and you've got the basics for getting a quick, healthy, and easy meal on the table.

You'll notice that some of these recipes call for spice mixes. Not only do spices make your food more flavorful, they also are loaded with health benefits on their own. I always like to get organic spices, but good spices aren't cheap. An easy way to save money is to buy the organic bulk spices at the store and only buy what you need. In the long run, you save money and your spices stay fresher.

Here are some of the most versatile recipes that I use for quick dinners. There are several websites and eBooks that have other great ideas. I've recently discovered New Leaf Wellness. They have many great recipes, shopping lists, and extremely affordable e-

Books. Having some meal plans together for the holidays can free your mind so you can relax and spend your time focusing on other things.

You can also save money by purchasing organic meats at your local Costco. They have organic grass-fed hamburger, organic whole chickens, chicken breasts, thighs, and legs. You'll also find some bags of organic frozen veggies. This allows you to prepare recipes in bulk at more affordable prices.

Because so many of us work, the crock-pot is a great tool to use to maximize your time. Here are a couple of my favorite recipes that I've discovered:

#1 - Salsa Chicken
(Remember to double the recipe if you'd like some for the freezer)

Ingredients:

1½ lbs. boneless, skinless chicken breasts. *I think chicken thighs would work just as well in this recipe if that's what you have on hand.*
2 cups salsa (I used a small jar of Whole Food's Organic Salsa for a single recipe)
Juice of ½ of a lime

Season with this:

DIY Taco Seasoning
(Season liberally, and store remainder for another time
– Tip – DIY Seasonings make a great holiday gift)

Ingredients:

2 Tbs. chili powder
1 Tbs. onion powder
1 Tbs. garlic powder
1 ½ tsp. coconut sugar
1 Tbs. ground cumin
2 tsp. sea salt, or to taste

2 tsp. paprika
2 tsp. dried oregano
½ tsp. crushed red pepper flakes (or to taste)
Optional: Cilantro or diced green onion for garnishing, ½ cup frozen Organic Corn, Cooked Rice, 1 can Black Beans (rinsed and drained), Sliced Avocado, Guacamole, Chopped Romaine Lettuce, Shredded Cheese, Salsa, and Sour Cream.

Method:

Place chicken in the crock-pot and season with your DIY Taco Seasoning Mix. *I like making my own seasoning mix with organic spices, but if you can find a good organic blend that is pre-mixed, then by all means use that.* Spoon salsa over seasoned chicken and cook in crockpot on low for approximately 6 hours.

If you'd like to add a can of rinsed and drained black beans, or ½ cup of organic frozen corn, add these ingredients to crock-pot one hour prior to the end of cooking time.

At end of cooking time, shred chicken, squeeze ½ the lime and stir with contents. Top with optional toppings of your choice such as cilantro, green onions, shredded cheese, guacamole, chopped avocado, additional salsa, or sour cream.

This recipe can be used in multiple ways. You can make some rice and create your own burrito bowl and top it with some shredded lettuce and more salsa. The mixture makes a great filling for tacos or burritos, and works well as a topping for nachos. It's also a wonderful topping for a baked potato, and leftovers can even be used to make Chicken Tortilla Soup. Leftovers can be frozen and pulled out to be reheated and used at another time.

#2 – Pulled BBQ Chicken with Slaw Topping

Ingredients:

3 to 4 pounds boneless skinless chicken thighs, or a mix of thighs and breasts

1 large onion, diced

2 (or more) cloves garlic, minced

2 tsp. smoked or regular paprika

2 tsp. sea salt

Freshly ground black pepper

1½ cups barbecue sauce (store-bought or homemade), plus more for serving. (*Check the ingredients carefully on the sauce you buy in the store for things like high fructose corn syrup or "natural" flavorings. Find ones with whole food ingredients with the least amount of sugar, or see the recipe below for a great homemade barbeque sauce that is simple to put together.*)

Method:

Salt and pepper chicken and place in crock-pot. Pour the barbeque sauce over the chicken and cook on low for approximately 6 hours. When chicken is finished, use two forks to shred finely.

You can serve this with gluten-free buns, slaw, avocado, and extra barbecue sauce on the side. You can refrigerate for up to 5 days or freeze for up to 3 months.

DIY BBQ Sauce

Ingredients:

½ Tbs. olive oil

¼ medium onion, diced

1 clove garlic, minced

1 Tbs. tomato paste (I like the organic tomato paste in the jars by *Jovial*)

½ tsp. cumin

1 (8-ounce) can tomato puree or sauce (I used a jar of *Jovial's organic diced tomatoes*)

2 Tbs. coconut sugar

1 Tbs. organic raw apple cider vinegar (I used the *Bragg's* brand)

1 Tbs. molasses

2 tsps. gluten-free Worcestershire sauce (I used *The Wizards* organic gluten-free Worcestershire sauce)

1 tsp. dijon or brown mustard

1 tsp. salt

A few dashes hot sauce (optional)

Freshly ground pepper

Method:

Heat a splash of olive oil in a medium saucepan over medium heat. Add the onions and cook until soft, about 5 minutes. Add the garlic and cook for another minute or two.

Reduce the heat to low and mix in the tomato paste and cumin. Add the tomato puree and all remaining ingredients. Stir until combined and simmer for 5 to 10 minutes, until thickened to your liking. Taste and adjust salt, pepper, or other seasonings as you see fit.

Transfer the sauce to a blender or use an immersion blender to blend until smooth. Add more water, a tablespoon or two at a time, if you prefer a thinner sauce.

Broccoli Carrot Cole Slaw with Lime Dressing

Ingredients:

½ head green cabbage, cored and shredded

1 bag broccoli and carrot slaw (organic)

1 large bunch cilantro, leaves roughly chopped (organic)

2-3 limes, juiced (about ⅓ cup)

⅔ cup avocado oil

1 to 2 tsps. coconut sugar
Sea salt and freshly ground pepper

Method:

Shred the cabbage finely using a chef's knife or a food processor's shredding blade. In a very large bowl, toss together the
shredded cabbage with broccoli and carrot slaw mix and chopped
cilantro.

Whisk together the lime juice, oil and sugar. Toss with the slaw,
and season generously with salt and pepper.

Best served within a day or two, cold from the fridge, but you
can refrigerate it for up to 3 days or until it loses its crispness.

#3 - Roast Chicken in the Crock-Pot

Ingredients:
1 (4 -5 lbs.) whole roasting chicken
3 tsp. sea salt
1 tsp. regular or smoked paprıka
1 tsp. onion powder
½ tsp. dried thyme
1 tsp. Italian seasoning
½ tsp. black pepper
½ tsp. cayenne pepper (optional)
4 whole garlic cloves (optional)
1 yellow onion, quartered (optional)
lemon wedges (optional)

Method:

Grease the inside of a 5-quart or larger crock-pot with a bit of olive oil, coconut oil, or ghee.

Combine the spices. You can do this ahead of time, label it, and place in a small sandwich bag or empty spice shaker to save time.

Rub the chicken with the dry ingredients, inside and out, and place the chicken in the crockpot, breast side down.

If desired, place onion, garlic, or lemon wedge inside chicken cavity (optional).

DO NOT ADD WATER. Cook on high for 4-5 hours, or 8 hours on low.

The chicken should be so tender it will fall off the bone. You can have this with dinner with a steamed vegetable, mashed sweet potatoes, or a big green salad. You can use the leftovers in salads, sandwiches, or wraps, or in a fast veggie stir-fry for a little protein. Save the carcass and bones and you can make a great chicken and veggie soup. Don't have time to deal with soup making right now? Put the carcass/bones into a big zip-lock bag and put it in the freezer to pull out at another time. You can also chunk up the leftover chicken and freeze the leftovers for another recipe later.

#4 - Black Bean and Sweet Potato Chili

Ingredients:

1Tbs. grass-fed butter or ghee

1 medium onion, chopped

1 red pepper, chopped

4 garlic cloves, minced

2 tsp. sea salt

2 large sweet potatoes, peeled and cut into ½ inch cubes

2 jars (15 oz.) diced organic tomatoes*

2 cans (15 oz.) of organic black beans, rinsed and drained*

1 Tbs. cumin

1-2 Tbs. chili powder

1 Tbs. cocoa powder

Optional: 1 cup chopped cilantro leaves (for garnish), 1 diced fresh jalapeno, squeeze of lime

Method:

Heat butter in pan and sauté onions, garlic and red pepper until soft (about 5 minutes). Add this mixture and remaining ingredients to the slow cooker and cook on low for 6 hours. Garnish with cilantro and squeeze of lime if desired prior to serving.

*To reduce exposure to BPA (Bisphenol A) always make sure you purchase tomato products in glass jars and look for beans in cans marked BPA-free, or cook your own beans and freeze them ahead of time for when you want to make this recipe.

#5 – Hamburger Stew

Ingredients:
1 pound ground beef
1 small chopped onion
1 cup chopped carrots
1 cup chopped celery
2 cloves minced garlic
2 cups chopped potatoes
1 15-ounce jar of diced tomatoes
2 tsp. gluten-free Worcestershire sauce (I use *The Wizards* organic gluten-free Worcestershire sauce)
4 cups water, beef broth, or a combination of the two. (If you use water, you will need more seasonings)
½ - 1 tsp. of various spices - oregano, basil, thyme, garlic powder, onion powder, paprika or other herbs. I also like adding red pepper flakes for flavor. Feel free to season to your personal preferences.
Salt and Pepper – Needs a good amount of salt in my opinion

Optional – mixed organic frozen vegetables (green beans, peas, corn), organic ketchup for additional flavoring.

Method:

Brown the ground beef in a medium fry pan, and drain excess fat. Place potatoes, carrots, celery, onions, and minced garlic in crock pot in that order. Top with cooked ground beef. Add tomatoes, liquids and spices. If you'd like to make this a vegetarian stew, simply replace the hamburger with a couple cans of beans and use vegetable stock. Cook on low for 8-10 hours, or on high 4-6 hours.

#6 - Meatloaf

Ingredients:

1 pound ground beef or ground turkey
1-2 grated carrots
1 onion diced
2 cloves minced garlic
1 egg
⅔ cup ketchup (save some for brushing on the top of the meatloaf)
¼ cup milk or milk alternative (I use almond milk)
⅔ cup dried bread crumbs, saltines or crackers (crushed), or oatmeal for binding – I use dried gluten-free bread or gluten-free oats
1 tsp. gluten-free Worcestershire sauce (I use *The Wizards* organic gluten-free Worcestershire sauce)
Salt and Pepper for Seasoning

Method:

In a bowl, mix the ground meat, salt, pepper, onions, garlic, and grated carrots and mix together. Add in the wet ingredients – ketchup (reserve some for brushing on top of meatloaf), milk,

Worcestershire sauce, and egg. Once incorporated, add in the dried bread, oatmeal, or cracker crumbs. Mix together.

You can choose to either form the mixture into a large loaf and bake in a lightly oiled bread loaf pan, or I have some silicone muffin cups that I fill for individual portions. I lightly oil the silicone baking cups to prevent sticking. I would recommend not baking them in the regular muffin tins, as cleanup is a bit tedious. Take a silicone pastry brush and brush the top of the meatloaf with the remaining ketchup.

For a large loaf, bake in your oven at 350 degrees for approximately 1 hour. I cover my meatloaf pan with a sheet of parchment paper and remove it about half way through the baking time. If you're cooking in the muffin cups, it takes approximately 35 to 40 minutes. I like to freeze my meatloaf once it is cooked, and I find it easy to double the recipe and make two – one for now and another for later.

#7 – Indian Dal Soup with Mixed Veggies
Ingredients:
1 lb. chana dal (split chickpeas) or toor dal (split yellow lentils)
2 medium onions, diced
6 cloves of garlic, minced
1 Tbs. ginger, minced
15 ounce jar of diced tomatoes
4 cups vegetable broth (low sodium or homemade)
4-5 cups water or more vegetable broth (more or less to thin as desired)
2 Tbs. cumin seed
1 tsp. roasted coriander powder (or regular)
1/4 tsp. tumeric powder
2 tsp. black mustard seeds

After dal is finished cooking add:

3 cups mixed frozen vegetables or other mixed diced vegetables

1 tsp. roasted cumin

1-2 Tbs. coconut sugar

3/4 tsp. Herbamare or salt to taste

fresh ground pepper to taste

1/2 bunch of organic cilantro, chopped

Method:

Pick over the dal/lentils and remove any discolored ones or stones. Rinse thoroughly and drain.

Place ingredients into slow cooker, except for frozen vegetables and additional spices and cook on low 10 hours, or high 7-8 hours. You can also cook this overnight and add the additional vegetables and seasonings the next day.

When the lentils are soft and breaking apart, add the vegetables and seasonings and let this cook for another 30 minutes or so. Taste test and adjust seasonings if necessary. Serve over rice and garnish with fresh cilantro.

The *Zen* Days of Christmas

On the **Eighth Day** of Christmas, My Health Coach Gave to Me:

Eight Gifts for Giving

Gift giving shouldn't be a choice between your peace of mind or your financial well-being. Often, it's those simple, thoughtful gifts that you've put some imagination into that mean the most. It doesn't even have to be a gift that requires purchasing anything. In today's world, people are short on time, and I bet you have something to offer to the people on your list that they would love.

That young family with little kids would probably love a date night, so give them a gift certificate for an evening out where you babysit their children.

For those elderly neighbors, I suggest things like bringing them a hot meal, shoveling their walks when it snows, or raking leaves in the fall. Or maybe it's as simple as inviting them over for a cup of coffee and some freshly baked cookies.

Maybe you're a whiz at the computer. There are many people who would love an hour of your time to show them how to install software, learn how to Skype or format a Word or Excel document.

Another great way to give gifts is to give gift certificates from the local vendors that take care of you throughout the year. If you have a great hairdresser or manicurist who is trying to grow their business, give one of your friends a gift certificate for a discount on an appointment. Do you have a great massage therapist or coach that you love? Give your friends a certificate for their services.

Another thing to consider is that there are many online businesses on the web, and almost all of them offer some sort of a free opt-in for joining their email lists. If you've found some great information online, download one of their freebies and print it off for a friend. If you know the interests of the people on your gift list, you can no doubt find something to introduce to them that they would enjoy.

Below, I've put together some other ideas for gifts giving that you might want to consider that can be purchased to help you with your holiday shopping:

#1 – Adult Coloring Books

There's a new hobby that many people are picking up, and I personally think it's brilliant. They have beautiful, detailed adult coloring books in all kinds of lovely designs. Coloring gives people's brains a chance to relax and it allows their creativity to kick in.

It's also something you can do with friends or family. Going out to dinner, and you know the wait is going to take some time? Take a coloring book, some crayons or colored pencils to the table and pass out a page for everyone to work on while they visit and wait for their food. Certainly beats watching everyone staring at electronic devices. A gift of a coloring book with some colored markers, pencils, or crayons makes a great gift.

#2 – Books

If you've read a great book that you enjoyed, chances are your friends would love it as well. A book with a note to that person about why you chose this book for them would make a lovely gift all on its own. You can also include a beautiful bookmark, and you've got a gift that anyone can appreciate.

Is the person planning an exciting trip to somewhere new? A travel book describing that destination makes a thoughtful gift, and if they are heading somewhere warm and sunny, think of including a quality sunscreen (I love the Badger brand sunscreen), some sun-blocking lip balm, a water bottle, or possibly a fun new hat or beach towel. Or, if they plan on skiing over the holidays, maybe some hand warmers, a nice scarf, a warm hat, or pair of gloves would make a wonderful and much-appreciated gift.

For the person who loves to cook, buy them a popular cookbook along with some wooden spoons, dishtowels, hot pads, or a cute little kitchen timer.

For the teachers on your list, I'd like to suggest some great books from my face reading mentor, Jean Haner. Her books, *The Wisdom of Your Child's Face* or *Your Hidden Symmetry* would make fascinating reading for those teachers who deal with the various faces and personality types of children on a daily basis.

For the older people on your list, large-print books or audio books would be a much-appreciated gift.

Inspirational books that spiritually inspire from all the Hay House Radio authors (www.hayhouse.com) make wonderful gifts and during the holidays they offer great deals.

Books for children are good choices for the kids on your list. Last year I bought *Goodbye Bumps* written by Wayne Dyer's daughter, Saje Dyer, and my grandchildren had me read it to them over and over again. Or, if you're a grandmother like I am, Mary Hansen Freund and Jane Freund's book *Grandma, Does My Moon Shine Over Your House* is a great way to connect with those special grandchildren that live in another location. *Pete the Cat – I Love My White Socks* by James Dean and several other Pete the Cat books are ones that are quite popular. Another book that was well received by my own grandchildren was *Marsupial Sue* by John Lithgow, which came with a CD and a song that they enjoyed learning.

If the person on your list owns a Kindle, consider giving them a Kindle or Amazon Gift card so that they can pick out the books they would like to read, which quite possibly might be the best way to go with the teens on your gift giving list.

#3 – Technology Gifts

People who use technology might enjoy the following gifts:

Orange Tinted Glasses – These rather wacky-looking glasses might help that techie in your life get a better night's sleep. Studies have indicated that blue light coming from all of our electronic devices, especially in the evening hours, can inhibit the body's production of melatonin, a hormone we produce that aids in helping people fall asleep. Orange-tinted glasses filter out this light and could be helpful in regulating the body's circadian rhythm so that you still produce the melatonin necessary for a good night's sleep. You can find these glasses for around $10 on the Internet.

Wipebooks – My son actually told me about these, and I think they're brilliant. These are little notebooks that take the idea of a dry erase board to a notebook. You can brainstorm with each other on these, and take pictures of the information or scan the page. You can then erase the contents to use for another day. What a great way to save a few trees on the planet.

#4 - Personal Care Products

So many of our personal care products contain toxic ingredients. Our skin absorbs these chemicals and for those individuals that are sensitive, these products can trigger not only skin issues, but can impact their health as well. A couple of years ago I developed some allergies to skin care products, and had to find natural ways to care for my skin. I started using natural products such as coconut oil, essential oils, lemons, avocados and honey. Before long, I was making my own lotion bars and lip balm. What I have discovered is that it is actually quite easy and economical to make your own products.

You can purchase glass containers at <u>www.aromatools.com</u> and make these products to give as gifts to your friends. Or, you can purchase some of the ingredients and creatively package them in a

DIY package. Include some recipes and containers and they're set to make some of these products on their own. Or, if you'd like, you can make the products yourself for your friends for gift giving. Here are few of my favorite personal care products that my friends enjoy receiving as gifts:

Lip Gloss

Ingredients:
4-5 Tbs. of organic castor oil. (Use 5 tablespoons of oil if you prefer a softer gloss, and 4 tablespoons if you would like a firmer gloss)
1 Tbs. beeswax pellets
2 tsp. honey
20 drops peppermint, spearmint or orange essential oil (optional)
¼ to ½ tsp. of powdered beet root for color (optional). Note – the more beet root powder you add, the darker the color will be.

Method:
I take a small wide-mouth glass jar and to this add the oil, honey, and beeswax. I then place this jar into a small saucepan filled with simmering hot water and stir the mixture until everything is melted and liquid. Before removing from the heat, stir in the beet root powder if you're adding this in, and stir until the liquid mixture looks completely incorporated.

Remove from the heat and add the essential oil (if desired). Set the jar in an ice water bath and stir rapidly with a small whisk or spoon until the mixture resembles a thick frosting. It will be pale yellow unless you have added the beet root for color.

Spoon the mixture into storage containers and cap. Let the mixture set for 2 hours prior to use. No refrigeration is required, but for maximum freshness and taste, please use within 1 year.

Lotion Bars

Ingredients:

1 cup coconut oil

1 cup shea butter, cocoa butter or mango butter (or a mix of all three butters equal to 1 cup)

1 cup beeswax pellets (you can add an extra ounce or two if you want a thicker consistency, which leaves less lotion on the skin when used)

Optional: Vitamin E oil to preserve (approximately 1 tsp.)

Essential oil of choice (approximately 40-50 drops)

(I like doTerra essential oils because of their quality. Lavender essential oil and peppermint essential oil work well. I also like doTerra's On Guard essential oil in the winter, as it is anti-bacterial and anti-viral. doTerra's Deep Blue or Wintergreen are great essential oil additions for people who have arthritis.)

Method:

Combine all the ingredients (except for the essential oils if using) in a quart-size, wide-mouth glass mason jar, and put the jar in a saucepan with 1 inch of water. Stirring occasionally over medium heat, stir until the ingredients are melted and smooth. I designate one jar specifically for this purpose, as this makes cleanup much easier.

Remove jar from heat and add the essential oils, stirring until incorporated. Carefully pour the liquid into the molds and place in your refrigerator to cool and harden. There are many silicone baking molds or ice cube trays available for purchase, and these work really well for making lotion bars. In fact, I bought some silicone ice cube trays recently at IKEA and I use these to make my lotion bars. Or you can also use a mini muffin pan.

Allow the lotion bars to cool completely before attempting to pop out of the molds.

Epsom Salt Bath Soak

Ingredients:
2 cups of Epsom salts
½ cup baking soda
2-3 drops of a quality lavender essential oil (optional)

Method:
Place this mixture in a glass jar along with these instructions:

Add these ingredients to a warm bath and soak for 15 to 20 minutes. Do this 2-3 times weekly. Epsom salts relax the body and provide the essential mineral, magnesium, which is necessary for optimal relaxation, digestion, cleansing and health.

I think it is nice to include a candle or a relaxing CD with this gift, or a dry skin brush with instructions on dry body brushing.

#5 – Foods

Healthy foods are something that every person will use, and below I've listed a couple of suggestions for ways to give this gift.

The Fruit Basket – Compile your own organic fruit baskets for family and friends. This is something that I have yet to find pre-made in the stores. Usually the stores will have fruit baskets, but it is difficult to find an organic fruit basket. Find some large baskets or plastic tubs and fill them with some quality organic fruit. Buy a roll of cellophane wrapping paper, gather it around the basket and fruit and tie on a festive bow. Or simply find a beautiful basket and add some red or green shredded paper and nestle the fruit in the basket.

The Smoothie Basket – Gather up some items that you enjoy in your smoothies and put these in a basket. You might find some organic nuts, a sack of Hemp Seeds, a package of medjool dates, a sack of goji berries or other superfoods, a jar of nut or seed butters, a jar of raw, unfiltered local honey, or a container of your favorite plant-based organic protein powder. Put in a Shaker Cup, a couple of your favorite recipes, and you've got a healthy and thoughtful gift that lets someone start out the New Year with a few healthy essentials.

Spice Mixes – Consider making some healthy spice blends for gift giving. Many of the packaged store-bought mixes contain ingredients that contain ingredients that such as MSG (which can trigger health concerns for many people), anti-caking ingredients, and other additives. Buy the spices for a couple of these mixes and package them in spice jars. Hint, if you have a local restaurant supply store or an IKEA locally, you can find containers rather inexpensively, and if you purchase your organic spices in bulk, you can save money as well. The Wellness Mama has some great DIY spice blend recipes on her site if you need some ideas.

(http://wellnessmama.com/4430/homemade-spice-blends/)

Consider pairing this gift with some of your favorite recipes that call for these mixes.

Herbed Butter – If you're going to someone's home, a thoughtful hostess gift is always appreciated, and this is one that takes very little time.

Herbed Butter

Makes about 1/2 cup (equivalent of 1 stick)

Ingredients:

½ cup (1 stick) organic unsalted butter, softened to room temperature

¼ cup finely chopped mixed herbs (such as basil, thyme, sage, pars-

ley, dill, chives, tarragon, oregano, marjoram or rosemary)
1 tsp. coarse sea salt
1 tsp. freshly ground black pepper
A general rule of thumb for making herb butters is for every cube of butter (½ cup, or ¼ pound), use 1 Tbs. of finely chopped, fresh herbs; or 1 to 1½ tsp. of crumbled dried herbs; or 1/2 teaspoon of ground seeds (i.e. dill seed, fennel seed, etc.)

Method:

In a small bowl, combine all ingredients and mix until well incorporated. You can place the butter into silicone molds for fancy shapes, or simply place on waxed paper or parchment paper, shape into a cylinder or disk, and cover this with plastic wrap. If using dried herbs, let the mixture stand at room temperature for 2 hours to allow flavors to blend. If using fresh herbs, the mixture should be chilled for at least 3 hours. Herb butter will last approximately 2 weeks in the refrigerator and in the freezer for a few months.

#6 – Subscriptions

It's always fun to gift subscriptions to magazines for people in your life, and it is something that they will enjoy receiving month after month in the mail. Think about the interests of the people on your shopping list. Here are a few suggestions to get you started:

Men - The men on your list might enjoy *Popular Mechanics, Popular Science, Road and Track, Motor Trend, Consumer Reports, Hot Rod, Circle Track, Sports Illustrated, Handyman, Popular Photography, Golf, Field and Stream, Bicycling* – the choices are endless. What do they enjoy? There's probably a magazine that they would appreciate receiving.

Women – The women on your list might enjoy magazines like *Shape, Women's Health, Better Homes and Gardens, Self, Yoga, Woman's World, Cooking Light, Martha Stewart Living, Cook's Illus-*

trated, Taste of Home, Food and Wine, Clean Eating, Gluten-Free Living, the list is actually only limited by the interests of the women on your gift giving list. If the people on your list are interested in alternative healing, check out this website for additional ideas www.alternativesforhealing.com/natural-health-magazines

I love listening to Hay House radio, and they have subscriptions that allow you to revisit programs in their archive section to listen to again.

Children – Children LOVE getting mail. Since I don't live close to my grandchildren, packages sent to them are a way for us to keep in touch with one another throughout the year. And a magazine is something they can look forward to receiving all year. Here's some choices they might enjoy: *Ladybug, National Geographics Little Kids, Highlights, Zoobooks, BabyBug, Spider* – this list also goes on and on and there are magazines for just about any age group.

#7 – Kitchen Gadgets

If you have someone who is interested in cooking or has a kitchen, for that matter, they might enjoy some of the following kitchen gadgets:

- Spiralizer
- Lemon Zester or Lemon Juicer
- Microplane
- Oil Mister
- Silicone Lids (for covering dishes)
- Silicone Muffin Cups
- Fermentation Jars (for making fermented vegetables)
- Canning Funnel
- NutriBullet
- Food Dehydrator

- Microplane Herb Mill
- Kitchen Scale
- Yogurt Maker
- Meat Thermometer
- Cast Iron Pots and Pans
- A Chef's Knife
- Silicone Basting Brushes
- Vegetable Peelers (my favorite is one from IKEA)
- Steamer Basket
- Salad Spinner
- Glass Storage Containers and Storage Bowls
- Cooling Racks
- Parchment Paper,
- Parchment Paper Baking Cups
- Twine
- Nut Milk Bag
- Tea Strainers,
- French Press
- Tea Kettle
- Immersion Blender
- Crock Pot
- Pressure Cooker
- Silicone Strainer
- On the Pot Clips and Spoon Rests
- An Apron

Hopefully you can find something on this list of options that they might enjoy. A holiday box filled with a few odds and ends of things you use and appreciate the most in the kitchen is always a welcome and thoughtful gift.

#8 – Tools

Let's face it, things break and home repairs happen. Here's some items you could assemble for someone just starting out in life on their own:

- Screwdrivers
- Pliers
- Socket Set
- Crescent Wrench
- Hammer
- Measuring Tape
- Stud Finder
- Level
- Square
- Selection of Brads, Screws, and Assorted Hardware
- Partitioned Hardware Storage Container
- Duct Tape
- Electrical Tape
- Dry Wall Anchors
- Command Adhesive Hooks
- Picture Hangers
- 5 Gallon Bucket with Tool Sleeve, Tackle Box, or Soft-Sided Tool Bag

You can also give them a document that includes links to You Tube videos to walk them through simple home repairs. Check out the following Internet resources such as the *FixIt Home Improvement Channel, Hometime, This Old House,* or *DIY* to name but a few.

And most people would probably welcome the gift of a nice flashlight. In my corporate job I was the only woman in a department of men. The men I worked with used to tease me about women and their fascination with shoes. But to me, men seemed to have a fascination with flashlights. One year for Christmas, I went to the local hardware store and put together little survival kits for each of the men and included – you guessed it - flashlights.

Your Favorite Things

What have you discovered this year that you love? One of my best friends loves a really nice bed, and she sent me a lovely set of sheets as a thank you gift. I probably would never have discovered these wonderful sheets on my own, but because she found something that she loved, she was able to share this with me. So, while I have given you some ideas, don't forget that you know the people on your gift list better than anyone, and a gift from your heart that is given with love and appreciation can never go wrong. Happy gift giving, friends!

The *Zen* Days of Christmas

On the **Ninth Day** of Christmas, My Health Coach Gave to Me:

Nine Teas for Steeping

There's nothing more comforting than ending a long, hectic day with a lovely cup of tea. Herbal teas not only taste great, they have a wide range health benefits that can settle an upset tummy, help you sleep, and calm an active mind after a long day. Teas are also a great source of vitamins and minerals, and there's something very ceremonial about the entire ritual of making a cup of tea.

Teas also make great Christmas presents for friends and family, so think of including them on your gift-giving list. There are numerous cups, pots, mugs and tea infusers that come in a variety of price ranges. A personal tea mug with a tea strainer along with a box of your favorite herbal tea makes a wonderful gift. You could also bake a basket of healthy mini muffins and include a box of tea to accompany it.

Just as with our food, teas can be contaminated with things such as pesticides and GMOs, so look for these quality organic brands when choosing your teas: Numi, Traditional Medicinals, and Rishi Tea are good choices that should be available in many local natural or whole foods markets. Recently, I discovered a brand of teas online that I have given as gifts and would recommend checking out – Dovetail Organic Teas. Also, I've ordered organic teas from Mountain Rose Herbs and think their products are excellent as well. If you're considering using another brand of tea, do your homework and check to see that no other ingredients have been added to the teas. I would recommend using a stainless steel or glass tea strainer, and avoid the paper and material tea bags. Believe it or not, many of those fancy tea bags often contain plastics or bleaches; things you don't want to be consuming in your efforts to eliminate toxins from your foods. Online blogger, Vani Hari, The Food Babe, (www.foodbabe.com) has some great information on tea in her 8/21/2013 blog post – *Do you know what's really in your tea?*

Of course, as with any food or herb, not every tea is good for every body, and the medicinal properties of herbal teas may not be advisable for everyone, so please check with your health care provider if you have questions as to whether a specific tea would be right for you.

When it comes to teas, the options are endless, but I've listed a few of my personal favorites that you might want to consider over the holidays:

#1 - Peppermint Tea

The rich holiday food can often leave us with abdominal gas and bloating, and peppermint tea is a great remedy in reducing these unpleasant symptoms. If you have nausea (without vomiting), peppermint tea can help soothe the stomach. It can also be used to relieve muscle spasms. (Note - If you're pregnant, trying to get pregnant, or are breast feeding, it is advisable to avoid peppermint tea.)

If the holidays have you wanting to snack more, peppermint tea just might help control your appetite. Many turn to peppermint tea when they are suffering from a cold or flu, and its nutritional profile of calcium, manganese, copper, potassium, folate, and vitamins A, B, and C can help to boost the body's immune system.

However, if indigestion or heartburn are an issue for you, then it is best to avoid peppermint altogether. It is also advisable to check with your pharmacist if you're taking any prescription drugs just to be sure that peppermint tea (which contains menthol) won't react with your medications.

Nothing says Christmas more than the taste of peppermint. As you're enjoying your cup of peppermint tea, think about those candy canes that Santa gave you as a child, and enjoy this simple pleasure.

#2 - Ginger Tea

Used as a digestive aid, ginger can be used to curb nausea, vomiting or an upset stomach due to motion sickness. Ginger is also an anti-inflammatory, and can help reduce pain and stiffness for people who suffer from arthritis. This brew makes a powerful drink for those times when you have a cold, as it can help to open up airways and improve circulation.

According to James L. Wilson, ND, DC, PhD, in his book *Adrenal Fatigue: The 21st Century Stress Syndrome*, ginger is an adaptogen that helps modulate cortisol levels.

You can buy dried ginger tea, or make fresh ginger tea by simmering a piece of ginger root on the stove for 10 to 15 minutes. To this mixture, add some freshly-squeezed lemon juice and a little honey.

#3 - Chamomile Tea

A gentle, calming and sedative tea made from flowers, chamomile tea can be helpful for people who deal with insomnia or anxiety.

Chamomile tea can relax your digestive muscles and may be helpful if your digestive processes have become a bit sluggish. Or, if diarrhea is the issue, it may help you recover more quickly. This tea is also helpful if you should come down with a cold or fever, and can be used as a gargle for inflammation of the mouth.

Topically, it can help soothe the skin and is believed to be more effective at controlling the pain, itch, and inflammation of minor skin irritations than some of the popular hydrocortisone products on the market.

For herbal teas, it is suggested to allow the tea to steep for approximately 5 to 7 minutes to get the most health benefits.

#4 - Red Rooibos Tea

Roobios tea originates from South Africa where it is valued for its many health benefits. High in vitamin C and minerals, it is high in antioxidants which help ward off disease and slow the signs of aging.

Red rooibos tea has no oxalic acid and therefore it can be consumed by people who have kidney stones. It is also low in tannins, so people with sensitive digestive systems often tolerate it well.

It is also thought to improve heart health, support the immune system, provide allergy relief, support bone health, soothe colic symptoms, control blood sugar and calm certain skin conditions.

There are various conditions that may make consuming this beverage inadvisable, such as for chemotherapy patients. Since roobios has been shown in certain studies to exhibit some estrogenic properties, it should probably be avoided if you have a hormone sensitive cancer. Also avoid this tea if you have an existing kidney or liver condition.

#5 - Lemon Balm Tea

If the dark winter days have got you down, then lemon balm just might be the tea you need to try, as it can be helpful in lifting the spirits.

Got a cold sore, suffer from chronic fatigue, or have the shingles virus? Lemon balm is a great anti-viral. It is also known for assisting in concentration and focus. It may also be beneficial to people with Grave's disease, as it has been shown to slightly inhibit the thyroid stimulating hormone. Since it is considered safe for children, it can help prevent nightmares consumed prior to bed. This herb also makes a refreshing iced tea, and can be flavored with lemon or maple syrup.

#6 - Milk Thistle Tea

When consumed as a tea, milk thistle is a gentle liver cleanser. This mild tea can help the liver to regenerate and function at a higher capacity and assist in the production of bile, which can help our body digest fats. Other health benefits from milk thistle include lowering cholesterol and blood pressure, preventing gallstones, and providing antioxidants that slow the aging process.

#7 - Rose Hip Tea

I remember my mother brewing rosehip tea during the winter months when I was growing up. I thought it tasted great, and its light pink color was so pretty. Rosehips are the fruit of the rose plant and are a great plant source of vitamin C, which is important for the immune system, skin and tissue health and adrenal function. It's a great tea to consider adding to your winter routine to help bolster your immune system.

#8 - Hibiscus Flower Tea

Hibiscus flower tea has been shown to be as effective as some prescription drugs in lowering blood pressure. It also can lower high cholesterol and bolster the immune system, as it is also high in vitamin C.

Research studies suggest that hibiscus tea lowers the absorption of starch and glucose and speeds up the metabolism, so this tea might be helpful to those people who are trying to drop a few pounds.

#9 - Tulsi Tea

Also known as holy basil, Tulsi tea is known for its calming effect, as well as its ability to strengthen the body's immune system.

Tulsi tea contains powerful adaptogens that improve our body's ability to adjust to stress. Because of these agents, Tulsi tea can help restore balance to the mind and help relieve stress and tension on the nervous system.

Additional health benefits include supporting healthy vision, enhancing respiratory function, increasing metabolism, helping to support healthy blood sugar levels and supporting digestive health. It can refresh you when you feel tired, help with clarity of the mind, and even aid in supporting normal cholesterol levels.

The *Zen* Days of Christmas

On the **Tenth Day** of Christmas, My Health Coach Gave to Me:

Ten Fingers Posing

Getting through the holidays is a challenge for most of us on many different levels. Even if we take great care of ourselves, we can find times where we experience emotional upsets and imbalances in our life and the stress of the holiday season just seems to create additional turmoil.

Believe it or not, you always have access to something magical that can help you rebalance your emotional self. These magic wands have been with you since your birth. They are your ten fingers, and they hold the key to helping you through this holiday season. Combine the skills I'm about to share with you with your breathing exercises, and you have the power to regroup and rebalance anywhere at anytime.

Recently, I have been studying something called Jin Shin Jyutsu, an ancient self-healing modality that is based in the eastern philosophy of harmonizing the life energy in the body in the same way that all of nature is able to rebalance itself. This practice is all about getting to know yourself and bringing this knowledge back to readjusting your body with the flow of Universal energy.

Our physical bodies are highly sophisticated energetic vortexes that are meant to flow, move, and release. Unfortunately what happens all too often is that when we are emotionally triggered, because of social protocols, past emotional conditioning, beliefs, etc., we bottle up our emotions, express them in inappropriate ways, or stuff them back down. As a result, over time we can experience the physical manifestations of these emotions as disease in our bodies.

Each of our fingers has the ability to rebalance the body on both the emotional and physical levels. The process is as simple as holding your fingers and breathing. You can do this in the checkout line at the store, in a meeting at work, or while sitting in your car at the traffic light waiting for the signal to change.

Here's the basics of what to do: Hold each finger, one finger at a time, by wrapping all the fingers of your opposite hand around the finger. For instance, start with your right thumb, and wrap that thumb with all the fingers of your left hand. Simply hold that finger and take some nice easy deep breaths – I'd say a minimum of 3 breaths per finger, but I would suggest you hold each finger until you feel a sense of calm return. Then, switch hands, and hold your left thumb with your right hand, and repeat the process through each of your ten fingers.

Each of these fingers has a specific relationship to certain emotions, as well as the ability to strengthen specific areas of the physical body. I'm going to introduce you to each of these amazing digits and the magic you can unlock just by holding your fingers.

Meet Your Thumb and the Emotion of Worry

Do you keep going over the same worrisome thoughts in your mind? Are you depressed, obsessive, or anxious? Hold your thumb. Even the smallest of children recognize that the thumb has the ability to calm, reassure, and soothe. Many children suck their thumbs, but now that you're grown, you can simply hold your thumb.

The thumb is associated with the spleen and the stomach in the body. It's about digesting – not only our food, but our emotions as well. The thumb helps us connect with our compassion - both of ourselves and with others in our life.

Meet Your Index Finger and the Emotion of Fear

Fear is not a bad emotion. It actually helps keep us safe. If you're out in the woods and a bear starts to chase you, your fear will kick in, you'll get a shot of adrenalin, and you'd better run. That's how it's supposed to work, but in today's world, you're probably not likely to be chased by a bear.

Fearful thoughts can come up for us in life, and it's critical to be able to sort out the fear that is real, so that we can take appropriate action, and equally important to acknowledge that there are also fears that are unrealistic. Believe it or not, not every thought we think is true.

When fear comes up, holding your index finger can help you to tap into your inner wisdom and courage. This finger can allow you to trust in unseen forces that are always there, supporting and working things out in ways that we can't even begin to understand or comprehend. Fear is believed to be the root of all the other emotions and can actually block the healing of the physical body.

Holding the index finger supports the functions of the kidneys and the bladder in the body. These organ systems connect us back to our inner strength and stamina that function as our body's battery. The Chinese refer to this inborn strength and energy as your jing. It is believed that you are born with only a certain amount of jing, so you need to use it wisely – not on unfounded fearful thinking.

So on those occasions when those unrealistic fears surface, hold your index finger. Inhale courage and wisdom, and exhale fear.

Meet Your Middle Finger and the Emotion of Anger

Anyone that has been driving for any length of time has undoubtedly been the recipient of that nasty middle finger gesture that is so prevalent in our modern society. Is it any wonder that the middle finger conveys the emotion of anger?

Anger is an emotion that really gets a bad reputation. It is basically a call for change and frustration with what is. It can be expressed in a healthy fashion and a not so healthy expression. It isn't healthy to continually suppress anger and hold it in, but blowing up at others isn't the way to go either. Holding your middle finger can help you rebalance your frustrations and help you find productive ways to work with this emotion. It can allow you to use this energy to serve as a booster rocket to make much needed changes and find a new approach to something that isn't a good fit anymore. Anger should be looked at as a call to action to create improvement in a productive and controlled fashion.

Holding those middle fingers instead of directing anger towards others can calm you down.

This finger relates to the body's organs of the liver and the gallbladder. These organs also help with the body's ability to detoxify and aids in digestion. It is interesting to note that quite often as people embark on dietary detoxification protocols feelings of anger and frustration can come up for them during the process. Since the liver is the organ that serves as a filter for toxins, is it any wonder that as we detoxify the body that these stored emotions are released back into the system during this cleanup process?

So as you can see, that middle finger deals with a lot of toxicity and calls us to create changes that will have lasting benefits for us in our daily life. Hold that middle finger and thank it for bringing to your attention what needs to change and as you exhale, let go of the tension and feel the empowerment to move forward with confidence and strength.

Meet Your Ring Finger and the Emotion of Grief

Not everyone is going to be joyous during the holiday season. This time of year can often bring up feelings of sadness, loss, and grief. Many people are experiencing the grief of losing someone dear to them, and thoughts of the past often call us back to remembrances of pain or regret.

Not to minimize these emotions in any way, as they are necessary to the healing process, but holding the ring finger can help with these feelings. This finger can help us to release. Maybe we need to allow ourselves to release this pent-up emotion, and that's what we are designed to do. The point is, as grief comes up in our life, we should allow ourselves to cry and release. It's only when we can finally let go that we can begin the process of healing. As we release, we connect with that Divine love and support that is always there for us. We remember that while we may be separated from those we love physically, that the emotional connections, memories, and the love are eternal. That knowledge allows us to release the grief and experience our memories in a way where we can still feel those important connections, but with less pain. Instead we replace the pain with thoughts of love and gratitude for the times shared, the memories we have made, and for the lessons taught.

The ring finger is also known as the spirit finger, and holding this finger can bring you back to the flow of releasing and making room to receive again.

In the body, this finger relates to the lungs and the large intestine. These organs have the function of releasing and receiving in the body as well. The job of the lungs is to not only bring oxygen into the body, but to expel carbon dioxide. The large intestines are the final step in the digestion process, absorbing excess liquids and releasing waste products that the body needs to eliminate. Just as these organs are programmed to receive and to release, so are we designed to experience the emotion of grief. We are meant to release and express this emotion so that joy can return. Holding your ring finger can help you find this natural rhythm in your own life.

Meet your Little Finger and the Emotion of Joy

The little finger is all about harmonizing back to a state of balanced joy. If you go about your life where you are not honoring the call of your heart, you will find yourself lacking joy.

Discernment helps you to recognize what brings you joy in life. It can point out when you need to walk away from the toxic people, substances, or thoughts that are causing you stress and anxiety.

In the physical body, the little finger corresponds with the organs of the heart and the small intestine. The heart is protected in the human body by a sack, known as the pericardium. The pericardium keeps the heart from over expanding when blood volume increases and limits the movement of the heart. I often refer to this as the heart protector.

Emotionally, our heart should also have a heart protector that serves to discern those people who are safe to allow into our hearts, and those that we should keep out. The small intestines also serve a similar role in the body. It is the job of small intestines to sort out the nutrients that are needed by the body and to keep out those that should be eliminated.

Without the pumping of the heart, there is no blood, no life force, and without the proper nutrients, our body will wither and die.

Holding the little finger helps us to regroup and rebalance our heart, our joy, and our passion in life and can help us find our way back to a healthy state of joy that supports us as we learn the skill of discernment – what to let in, and what to keep out.

The *Zen* Days of Christmas

On the **Eleventh Day** of Christmas, My Health Coach Gave to Me:

Eleven Minutes Moving

So I've got to be really honest with you. This time of year, movement (a less charged word than exercise) gets more challenging for me. You see, my favorite way to move is to go for a walk outside. But I'm afraid I'm kind of a fair weather walker. I don't like it if it is too hot, too cold, too windy, if it's snowing or raining. And since I live in a state that experiences the four seasons, I'm faced with all of these distractions that nature throws my way. I have a cat that must take after me. She begs to go outside daily, but when I open the door to rain, snow, or extreme cold, she looks at me accusingly as if I have conspired against her and certainly must have some control over the weather.

This past year, I did a pretty good job of getting in a daily walk until the weather turned cold and the snow came. So now, I'm faced with the challenge of how to incorporate more movement in a way that is simple and quick. With all of our other obligations during the holidays, we're all challenged to find the time to get some exercise.

So that's why I've decided to implement the Eleven Minutes Moving philosophy to remind myself of my need to move on a daily basis.

The thought process is simple. Commit to moving a minimum of 11 minutes daily. That's all, and everything counts as movement, and bonus points if you do more than the 11 minutes.

You need something to use, such as a stopwatch, or even just a simple wind up kitchen timer can do the trick. It really isn't all that important if you track it or not – I just want movement in your awareness in everything you do.

Watching TV? The commercial break is your cue to get up and move and not sit back down until the program resumes.

Going shopping? Your job is to find a parking space as far away from the door of the store as possible and then to walk briskly into the store. Pretend they have a sale that is about to expire, and you want to get there quickly so that you can get a good deal.

Traveling by car? Take advantage of those stops at the rest area to do a couple of laps around the property before getting back into the car.

Traveling by air? Instead of just sitting there mindlessly waiting for your flight, staring at Facebook or checking your email, walk around the concourse while you wait. If you have your luggage, pull that along with you, as the added weight resistance from the luggage builds muscles.

Have a desk job? Set a reminder for each hour of the workday to get up and take a lap around the office. You can set appointment reminders that will go off to remind you to get up and take a break. Take the stairs instead of the elevator to and from work each day. If you have a question for someone in the building, take a walk and personally get up from your desk and go ask them instead of using emails, texts, or phone calls.

If you have kids, have dance breaks where you put on some lively music and dance around the living room with them. Kids know how to move, so watch them to see how it's done. Ask any mother of a young toddler how she gets her exercise, and she'll probably laugh at you. They pretty much go non-stop from one thing to the next, faster than Mom or Dad can keep up with their activities around the house.

Do you have a dog? Take the dog out for a walk. It's a great way to meet your neighbors, and if you won't walk for yourself, you probably would walk to keep your best friend happy and healthy.

Try Super Brain Yoga. There's a simple squat exercise that will not only get you moving, but might just make you smarter and calmer while you get in your daily 11 minutes moving. Known as Super Brain Yoga, this simple technique has been shown to enhance brain health in children with Attention Deficit Disorder (ADD), Attention Deficit Hyperactivity Disorder (ADHD), Down Syndrome, Alzheimer's, and other development challenges and cognitive delays.

Research conducted by Dr. Joie P. Jones of the Department of Radiological Sciences at the University of California uses the body's major acupuncture points – the earlobes, and the tips of the fingers to stimulate specific neuropathways in the body. According to Dr. Jones, after doing the exercise, an EEG scan shows the synchronization of both the right and left hemispheres of the brain.

The process is outlined below:

- Face East. For the elderly, face North. The Chinese 5 Elements believes that specific energies govern each of the directions. Younger people can handle change and growth more easily (East energy) than the elderly or ill who may need more of a restorative energy (North energy.)
- Remove jewelry and connect your tongue to the roof of your mouth, leaving it there throughout the exercise.
- Take your left hand, cross your upper body to take hold of your right earlobe with thumb and forefinger. Make sure that the thumb is in front.
- Now take your right hand across your upper body to take hold of your left earlobe. Again, make sure that the thumb is in front. At this point you're pressing

both earlobes simultaneously. Make sure your left arm is close to your chest and inside your right arm.

- Inhale through your nose and slowly squat.
- Hold your breath and exhale as you start making your way back up to a standing position.
- Repeat this squatting action 14 times. Continue to hold your earlobes and to keep your tongue touching the roof of your mouth throughout the exercise.

If you're interested in reading more about this process, please visit www.superbrainyoga.com.au

For some folks, mobility is an issue. People who have issues with walking might consider getting some small hand weights or exercise bands. Stretching exercises can also be helpful to relax muscles, increase flexibility, and reduce pain, and simply standing up and sitting back down can provide great exercise.

So regardless of whether you're a yogi, a runner, a walker, or someone who is a professional couch potato, there's a variety of ways to move more in life. I encourage you to find what works for you and find daily ways to simply move more.

The *Zen* Days of Christmas

On the **Twelfth Day** of Christmas, My Health Coach Gave to Me:

Twelve Oils for Healing

Over the last few years, I have changed the way I take care of my minor aches and pains. I haven't taken an over-the-counter remedy in the past three years. What I have discovered instead are essential oils. I use these oils to clean my home, make my own personal care products, rub on my stomach for digestive issues, and create compresses for headaches or aching backs. To be perfectly honest, I don't know what I did before I started using these oils. In a word, they have changed how I take care of my family and my health, and I'm extremely grateful to have discovered them.

An essential oil is a liquid that is generally distilled (most frequently by steam or water) from the leaves, stems, flowers, bark, roots, or other components of a plant. Because of this process, the healing compounds from these plants are super concentrated, so just a few drops provide powerful healing properties.

Essential oils can be used by combining them with a carrier oil such as coconut oil, almond oil, apricot kernel oil, or grapeseed oil and rubbing them directly on the skin; the bottoms of the feet is often the best and safest place to apply. They can also be inhaled through the use of an essential oil diffuser, and some can used in personal care products.

There are many brands of essential oils on the market. I'm not trying to promote the quality of one brand of oil over the other, but I would suggest that you are as diligent in choosing an essential oil as you would be in choosing other foods or herbs, as quality does matter.

The prices and quality of essential oils can vary depending on the rarity of the plant, the country of origin, growing climate, quality control standards of the various distillers, and the amount of oil that is produced. I personally use doTerra oils, but have friends that use Young Living oils, and they love them as well

For the purposes of this book, since I'm speaking of my own personal experiences and the oils I use and love, I'll be presenting information on the doTerra oils.

As with any plant-based or herbal consumable, essential oils may not be appropriate for everyone, so if you have any existing health conditions, are pregnant or nursing, or are taking prescription medications, it's always best to consult with your health care provider prior to using them to be certain you will not have any unwanted side effects.

I'd like to introduce you to a few essential oils that I personally use and love:

#1 – Lavender

Lavender is one of my favorite oils and is known as the calming essential oil. Lavender essential oil is the one to use to relax and prepare for sleep.

This oil is great at creating a peaceful and calming atmosphere, which is why it is wonderful to diffuse in your home or your bedroom. I also like to add a couple of drops in my bath water, along with some Epsom salts for a relaxing soak in preparation for bed. Who couldn't use a little more of this peace and relaxation during the holidays?

It's also a great oil to have in the kitchen for minor burns and wounds. I've burned my fingers on more than one occasion, and lavender oil is great at taking the pain away quickly. A few years ago, I got into a struggle with a garbage can in my yard and ended up banging up my arm as a result. Lavender oil came to my rescue and quickly soothed the pain.

#2 – Peppermint

If there is a smell that we often think of in association with Christmas, it's the smell of peppermint. Peppermint essential oil is a great one to reach for if you're suffering from nausea. It can also increase energy and is great at easing headaches, so if your energy needs a boost, consider turning to some peppermint essential oil for a natural pick-me-up. You can also apply peppermint oil to the bottoms of the feet to reduce fevers.

#3 – Frankincense

Another oil that makes you think of Christmas is frankincense. After all, this is one of the essential oils given to baby Jesus by the Three Wise Men. Frankincense has been considered to be more precious than gold and revered by royalty throughout history.

When I first started using essential oils, I knew I wanted to try frankincense, as it is an anti-viral, anti-bacterial, and anti-fungal essential oil. I remember someone once telling me – "When in doubt, get the frankincense out." I use this oil in healing any skin issue and it is a wonderful oil to put in any skin care product.

Frankincense is high in sesquiterpenes, which have been studied for the potential to cross the blood brain barrier and oxygenate the pineal and pituitary glands.

Adding a few drops of frankincense oil to a hot bath works great to relieve stress and fight anxiety. Some people believe that the fragrance of frankincense can increase your intuition and connection to spirit.

#4 – Breathe

No one wants to be sick with a cold over the holidays, but it can happen, and if it does, Breathe is a great blend of oils to have on hand. You can apply Breathe (combined with a carrier oil) topically to your neck and chest or rub on the bottoms of the feet to clear sinuses or help with congestion or a cough.

You can also diffuse this blend in water to help everyone in the house breathe easier. Breathe contains a combination of the following essential oils: laurel leaf (bay), peppermint, eucalyptus, melaleuca, lemon, and ravensara,

#5 – Melaleuca

Melaleuca, sometimes referred to as tea tree oil, is a great antimicrobial essential oil. The leaves of the melaleuca tree have been used for centuries by certain indigenous peoples to heal cuts, wounds, and treat skin infections. I've used this essential oil to treat cold sores, fungal infections, and skin rashes. It can also help in the treatment of acne. In fact, some studies indicate that is as effective as benzoyl peroxide, without some of the unwanted side effects such as red and peeling skin.

It's a wonderful oil to use in cleaning your home. I use a drop or two in water to wipe down countertops. If you have mold issues, melaleuca essential oil can be used to spray down the shower curtain, or you can add it to the washing machine or dishwasher.

#6 – DigestZen

If you experience digestive issues, this is an essential oil blend that you'll want to keep on hand. This is my go-to oil for upset stomachs. I take DigestZen with me when I travel, as sometimes eating out can aggravate digestive issues.

DigestZen contains ginger, peppermint, tarragon, fennel, caraway, coriander, and anise (all of these are known for their calming, anti-carcinogenic, anti-bloating and anti-intestinal spasm qualities). I rub it on my abdomen with some coconut oil at night – especially if dinner didn't agree with me. It helps me regulate my digestive system, and it's one oil that I'm never without. So if that holiday party leaves you feeling bloated and miserable, reach for the DigestZen.

#7 - Deep Blue

Deep Blue is another blend of essential oils specifically for aches and pains. It works wonders for muscle pain, arthritis, joint pain, and sprains. Definitely an oil that you'll want to keep around – especially if those 11 minutes moving were a little too much for you – Hah! Have it on hand if you overdo it shoveling snow or if hanging those Christmas lights left you feeling stiff and sore.

Deep Blue contains wintergreen, camphor, peppermint, blue tansy, german chamomile, helichrysum, and osmanthus. If you've got pain due to sprains or strains, this is an oil that you'll want to have around. They also make this in a lotion.

#8 - Wild Orange

It's no fun if you're feeling blue during the holidays, so if your mood could use a little lift, try diffusing some Wild Orange essential oil. A powerful cleanser and purifying agent, it's a great oil to consider adding to your winter routine, as it helps protect against seasonal and environmental threats by boosting your immune system.

Personally, though, I love it for the emotional and energetic boost it provides. Orange essential oil is known as the oil of abundance, and is believed to help open the mind and heart to the potential that exists all around us, encouraging us to accept and receive these blessings. After all, Christmas isn't all about giving. It is about learning to be a grateful recipient as well.

#9 – Lemon

Lemon essential oil is very handy for cleaning and degreasing. Got some pitch on your hands from the Christmas tree? Put a drop of lemon essential oil on it and it will come right off. It also works great to take those sticky labels off of glass jars.

I make a stain treatment for my laundry and a DIY carpet cleaning solution with this oil for when my cats "puke", as all cats do on occasion. I also like to add a few drops to my dishwater to help cut grease on dishes. A drop or two of this oil, added to water, works great as a cleansing soak for your vegetables and fruits. You can also put a few drops in a glass spray bottle and keep it on hand to clean and deodorize your cutting boards, and you can use it along with vinegar and water for general cleaning and deodorizing around the house.

You can put a drop in your drinking water to help with weight loss, boosting the metabolism, and detoxification.

If you feel the start of a cold, lemon essential oil can help with lymphatic drainage. Just combine a drop with some coconut oil and rub it on your neck. You can also make a great homemade cough syrup by combining a drop of lemon essential oil with some raw unfiltered honey.

And if that isn't enough, it smells great and will also help to boost your mood. So if cleaning your house this holiday season has you in a funk, break out that lemon essential oil and as Snow White says, just "Whistle While You Work".

#10 – OnGuard

If Christmas had a smell – other than peppermint, OnGuard would be that smell – at least to me. I love the spicy scent of this oil!

But don't let this lovely scent fool you. This is one powerful combination of essential oils that contains anti-viral, anti-bacterial, and anti-fungal properties. I keep this oil on hand specifically for the cold and flu season, and I like to think of it as my immune system supporter. I apply it daily as a defense against illness, and use it liberally if anyone gets sick.

I add a drop or two of this oil to a mixture of liquid castile soap and glycerin, and put it in one of those foaming hand soap dispensers.

Onguard is a wonderful oil to add to your essential oil diffuser during the winter months. My father is in an Assisted Living facility and he has an essential oil diffuser on his end table by his bed, and we diffuse this as a way to help protect him from viruses. It's been interesting to note that when people come into his room, they remark how great the room smells, but secretly I know that it goes beyond just a nice smell, it is doing important work to keep him healthy.

Onguard contains wild orange, clove bud, cinnamon bark, eucalyptus radiata, and rosemary.

#11 – Melissa

I've got to admit, this isn't an oil I use all the time, but it is one that I like to have on hand. I reach for Melissa if I feel a cold sore coming on. This oil is active against the herpes virus family. If you put some on the skin when you feel the first tingle, it will quite often stop the cold sore from developing at all.

In researching this oil, I also discovered Melissa can serve as a natural antidepressant, can support the respiratory system, works to calm the mind and relieves anxiety. Sounds like an oil that could be very handy to bring out over the holidays for a wide variety of reasons.

#12 – Whisper

Whisper is my all-time favorite essential oil blend for it's aroma. I use this for perfume because it just smells so good. If soft had a smell, it would be Whisper. This oil combines with each person's unique body chemistry to create a fragrance that is unique to that individual.

Whisper is a blend of wonderful essential oils - bergamot peel, ylang ylang flower, patchouli leaf, vanilla bean absolute, jasmine flower absolute, cinnamon bark, labdanum, vetiver root, hawaiian sandalwood, cocoa bean absolute, and rose flower essential oils in a base of fractionated coconut oil.

In addition to wearing it as a perfume, I like to diffuse this oil in my home. I also put some on a cotton ball and place it next to my vacuum cleaner bag. When I vacuum, it adds a lovely scent to the room.

This oil makes a wonderful gift along with an essential oil terra cotta necklace.

The *Zen* Days of Christmas

Closing Thoughts

I hope you have enjoyed the Zen Days of Christmas and that you're able to use some of these suggestions to help you navigate not only the holiday season, but to find your inner balance each and every day of the year.

As you grow in the awareness of what it takes for you, personally, to feel calm, balanced, and centered, you give not only to yourself, but also to others, the greatest gift each of us has to offer – the gift of your loving presence. Definitely a commodity that cannot be purchased in any store, and one that is most definitely a rare find in today's modern and fast-paced world.

Wishing you a holiday filled with peace, joy, and most of all love.

Merry Christmas!

About the Author

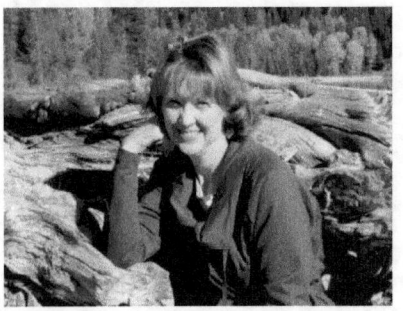

Carlene Snyder is a Certified Holistic Health Coach and graduate of the Institute for Integrative Nutrition. The mother of two grown children and three adorable grandchildren, she shares her life with her husband of 40 years and their three cats (her personal Zen teachers). Carlene owns and operates Zensational Health, located in Boise, Idaho. She can be reached at zensationalhealth@gmail.com.